GROW YOUNGER

Yes, you can prevent—and even reverse—the ravages of aging: wrinkles…high blood pressure…weight gain…aches and pains…memory loss. How? Through the amazingly simple and natural process of "youthing."

Our bodies are designed to live to at least 120 years, some say 140, all without drugs, surgery, or artificial elements. *Look Younger, Live Longer* blasts the myths of aging and offers a proven youthing plan like none you've ever seen or read. It costs practically nothing but time, and will give you immediate results, no matter what your current age!

The secret to growing younger is as easy as A, B, T—alpha, beta, and theta—brain wave patterns that make up the various stages of hypnosis. We actually experience hypnosis every time we daydream, which occurs three to four hours daily. To tap the fountain of youth, you simply need to take the daydream time that already exists and use it to strengthen your immune system. A strong immune system is the key to fighting old age.

Soon you can laugh at those who say, "You're not getting any younger." Everything you need to start turning back the clock is here, in *Look Younger, Live Longer.*

ABOUT THE AUTHOR

Dr. Bruce Goldberg holds a B.A. degree in Biology and Chemistry, is a Doctor of Dental Surgery, and has an M.S. degree in Counseling Psychology. He retired from dentistry in 1989, and has concentrated on his hypnotherapy practice in Los Angeles. Dr. Goldberg was trained by the American Society of Clinical Hypnosis in the techniques and clinical applications of hypnosis.

Dr. Goldberg has been interviewed on the Donahue, Oprah, Leeza, Joan Rivers, The Other Side, Regis and Kathie Lee, Tom Snyder, Jerry Springer, Jenny Jones, and Montel Williams shows; by CNN, CBS News, and many others.

Through lectures, television and radio appearances, and newspaper articles, including interviews in *TIME, The Los Angeles Times,* and *The Washington Post,* Dr. Goldberg has educated many people in the benefits of hypnosis. He has conducted more than 33,000 past life regressions and future life progressions since 1974, helping thousands of patients empower themselves through these techniques. His cassette tapes teach people self-hypnosis, and guide them into past and future lives. He gives lectures and seminars on hypnosis, regression and progression therapy, and conscious dying; he is a also a consultant to corporations, attorneys, and the local and network media. His first edition of *The Search for Grace* was made into a television movie by CBS. His third book, *Soul Healing,* is a classic on alternative medicine and psychic empowerment. Dr. Goldberg's column "Hypnotic Highways" appears in *FATE* magazine.

Dr. Goldberg distributes cassette tapes to teach people self-hypnosis and to guide them into past and future lives. For information on self-hypnosis tapes, speaking engagements, or private sessions, Dr. Goldberg can be contacted directly by writing to:

Bruce Goldberg, D.D.S., M.S.
4300 Natoma Avenue
Woodland Hills, CA 91364
Telephone: (800) KARMA-4-U or (800) 527-6248
Fax: (818) 704-9189
email: karma4u@webtv.net, Web Site: drbrucegoldberg.idsite.com

(Please include a self-addressed, stamped envelope with your letter.)

DR. BRUCE GOLDBERG

LOOK YOUNGER, LIVE LONGER

ADD 25 TO 50 YEARS TO YOUR LIFE, NATURALLY

1998
Llewellyn Publications
St. Paul, Minnesota 55164-0383, U.S.A.

FIRST EDITION
First Printing, 1998

Cover design by Tom Grewe
Cover photo supplied by Index Stock Photography,
    photograph by Melanie Carr
Editing and interior design by Connie Hill

Library of Congress Cataloging-in-Publication Data
Goldberg, Bruce, 1948–
    Look younger, live longer : add 20 to 50 years to your life, naturally / by Bruce Goldberg
        p. cm. --
    Includes bibliographical references and index.
    ISBN 1–56718–321–2 (pbk.)
    1. Longevity.   2. Aging.   I. Title.
RA776.75.G65   1998
612.6'8—dc21   97-32142
                                                                 CIP

Llewellyn Publications
A Division of Llewellyn Worldwide, Ltd.
St. Paul, Minnesota 55164-0383, U.S.A.

Printed in U.S.A.

ACKNOWLEDGMENTS

I would like to express my appreciation to Nancy J. Mostad, acquisitions and development manager for Llewellyn Publications, without whose interest in my work this relationship with Llewellyn would not exist. Words cannot express my gratitude to Carl Llewellyn Weschcke, president of Llewellyn Publications, for his encouragement and his interest in alternative medicine. He is most definitely a builder of bridges.

This book's final form would not be what it is without the assistance of my editor, Connie Hill. Thank you, Connie, for your kindness, professionalism, and helpful suggestions. I would also like to thank my patients for their participation and success at "youthing." Without their demonstration of the benefits of these natural techniques, this book would not have been possible.

OTHER BOOKS BY DR. BRUCE GOLDBERG

Past Lives—Future Lives
The Search for Grace: The True Story of Murder and Reincarnation
Soul Healing
Peaceful Transition: The Art of Conscious Dying
    & the Liberation of the Soul

Forthcoming

New Age Hypnosis
Protected by the Light: The Complete Book of Psychic Self-Defense
Time Travelers from Our Future
Astral Voyages: Mastering the Art of Soul Travel
Dream Your Problems Away: Techniques for Dream Empowerment
The Ultimate Truth: The Light at the End of the Tunnel
Lose Weight Permanently & Naturally
Custom Design Your Own Destiny
Sexual Bliss
Heaven Can't Wait

CONTENTS

NOTE TO THE READER

This book is the result of the professional experiences accumulated by the author since 1974, working individually with over 11,000 patients. The material included herein is intended to complement, not replace, the advice of your own physician, psychotherapist, or other health care professional, whom you should always consult about your circumstances prior to starting or stopping any medication or any other course of treatment, exercise regimen, or diet.

At times, the masculine pronoun has been used as a convention. It is intended to imply both male and female genders where this is applicable.

Some of the minor details in the case histories have been altered to protect the privacy of the author's patients. All of the names used, except those of the celebrities mentioned, have been altered. Everything else in these pages is true.

INTRODUCTION

Aging slowly allows us to enjoy life to the hilt, rather than expend our energies resisting Father Time. The very thought of growing old and the inevitable difficulties usually associated with aging depresses most people. Now science is on the threshold of showing us how aging can be prevented, or at least delayed.

By adopting a proactive lifestyle and utilizing the other recommendations presented in this book, high blood pressure, wrinkles, weight problems, aches and pains, heart problems, cancer, and other worries can be prevented or postponed. The result is a longer and more fulfilled life.

Look Younger, Live Longer presents both theory and specific techniques to deal with life's challenges associated with aging. I have drawn from the fields of gerontology (the study of aging), personal grooming, nutrition, exercise, biochemistry, and alternative medicine to present the most accurate and useful information available about improving and retaining vigor throughout life. Part I deals with the theoretical considerations of aging and how our body and mind provide us with natural methods to slow down the process.

My approach is holistic: all facets of life are necessary and work better together than they do alone. This book teaches you how to enjoy a longer and more fulfilled life, while raising your consciousness at the same time. I refer to this process as "youthing." Part II details simple and inexpensive steps to help you look younger and live longer.

We will see how our bodies are designed to live to be at least 120, or even 140. The average age to which Americans live today is only 75. By proper training and following nature's intent, it is not difficult to see how we can add 45 to 65 years to our lives. My estimate of 25 to 50 years is conservative!

This book is very different from the usual plethora of books on aging in that it presents an entirely natural approach. No drugs, surgery, or artificial elements of any kind are suggested. In some cases you will see how the aging process can actually be reversed. Scripts of self-hypnosis exercises to raise your consciousness are included in chapter 13. All of this culminates in a comprehensive youthing plan that is easy to apply and is like no other you have ever seen or read. It will cost practically nothing but time to implement and will give you immediate results.

We will discuss the "supernormals," people who live to be well over 100 while leading vigorous lives. Just think of these famous people from recent history: Bertrand Russell, George Bernard Shaw, Winston Churchill, Albert Schweitzer, George Burns, Pablo Picasso, Grandma Moses, Arturo Toscanini, Konrad Adenauer, Pablo Casals—these men and women retained their vigor and creativity well into their eighties and nineties, some even past the 100-year mark!

Butch Cassidy said to the Sundance Kid, "Every day you get older—that's a law." In the United States, it is estimated that at least 32,000 men and women are a hundred years old or older. More than ten percent of the population in America is over 65. If Butch Cassidy were alive today he might just have to eat his words.

Some animals are unusually long-lived. The Galapagos tortoise, for instance, can go on for well over 150 years, and may live into the beginning of a third century. Trees in the arid American West have endured for hundreds, even thousands, of years. In the mid-1950s, Edmund Schulman of the University of Arizona's pioneering Laboratory of Tree Ring Research found bristlecone pines in California that were nearly a thousand years older than the oldest known sequoias—until then rated the most ancient living things on earth.

To solve the problem of aging we need to look at DNA (deoxyribonucleic acid). This double-helix in the nucleus of every cell is the master molecule of all life. All genes and chromosomes are made up of this DNA.

DNA is millions and millions of years old—yet shows no signs of old age. As far as we know, DNA is the only organic substance in the universe that possesses the information to ensure its own virtual immortality. DNA has the unique ability to duplicate itself, again and again, almost without limit—as long as there are materials available from which it can manufacture new copies of itself.

Our DNA is passed on to our children and to their children through the mother's egg and the father's sperm. We may die, but our DNA survives. Do we use DNA to keep our species alive, or does DNA use us as hosts for its eternal survival?

Experts do not agree on what causes aging, and what, if anything, may be done about it. In fact, the standard cliché used to be that there seemed to be as many theories about aging as there were gerontologists. Despite this debate, gerontologists are beginning to show optimism and excitement about youthing.

This book surveys current gerontological research and theory, and explores the obvious question about the prospects of slowing down the advance of or even abolishing old age, and of significantly extending the vigorous years of our lives. We have already begun to harness DNA and its genetic code to our own ends. A final conquest of old age is in hand.

More people are beginning to understand and to believe that something can be done about the aging process, that as a species we are not forever doomed to undergo the ravages of senescence (aging). This realization has resulted in a number of new books about the aging process, and the appearance of new organizations devoted to aging research, such as the American Longevity Association (ALA), the American Foundation for Aging Research (AFAR), and the Fund for Integrative Biomedical Research (FIBER), as well as the work and support of the National Institute on Aging (NIA) itself.

The NIA has shifted its previous research emphasis from the pathology of old age to focusing on a healthy old age. We may already have the means to live out long lives and yet escape both physical and mental decrepitude, according to the U.S. government.

My purpose in writing this book is to present you with solid scientific and clinical evidence of what you can and cannot do to look younger and live longer naturally. Secondarily, the book will provide you with the means by which you can retard the "normal aging" process every single day of your life.

Preventive medicine and its analogs (nutrition, gerontology) have become important to the lives of millions of Americans. Another positive aspect of alternative health care has been the emphasis on the contribution of the mind to the state of one's health. The natural approaches presented here are simple and inexpensive measures that you can take to lead a better and longer life, with greater enjoyment and fewer illnesses. You will learn how to cope with today's stressful lifestyle, and at the same time retard the aging process.

I refer to this extension of life qualitatively as "youthing." My youthing program consists of managing:

- What you eat and drink.

- What you do with your body.

- What you do with your mind.

- Your environment and lifestyle.

I am a scientist, with degrees in biology and chemistry, dentistry and counseling psychology. Since 1974 I have worked hard in establishing an international reputation as an alternative medicine practitioner. Having published a dozen articles in scientific journals, I am well aware of the scientific method. My own professional reputation stands behind everything I do and write. My own case history will be presented in chapter 14 to illustrate that I practice what I preach.

The breakthroughs presented in this book cover a broad spectrum. Some of these are as follows:

- How to look younger immediately (chapter 8).

- How simple exercises will prolong your life (chapter 11).

- The "Antiviral Cocktail," first developed for AIDS, that can help increase your immune strength (chapter 10).

- The dietary key to reducing the cellular changes leading to old age, and an eating plan to help you use it (chapter 10).

- The nutritional keys you can use now to decrease the aging of your skin (chapter 10).

- Simple techniques to boost your brain power and improve memory and concentration (chapter 10).

- A simple method to significantly improve your sex life (chapter 12).

- A specific nutritional plan to take you off the danger list for cardiac problems (chapter 10).

- A simple exercise guaranteed to raise your consciousness and add many quality years to your life (chapter 13).

- A step-by-step plan to reprogram the internal computer that may be aging you prematurely (chapter 13).

By following these recommendations and simple techniques, I can assure you of a longer and happier life. Ignoring these suggestions will unquestionably result in a shortened, less healthy, and far less productive life. When it comes to youthing, it is clear that the biggest differences lie in the choices we make many times each day: decisions about what we will eat, how we move, how we treat ourselves, even what inner tapes we play as we drift off to sleep at night. Being around, enjoying life in 30, 40, 50 or 65 years means having a strong inner commitment to longevity, starting right now.

If you are 50 or so, you can expect to add 25 to 50 quality years to your life with this program. Those of you under 30 could see this figure swell to 45 to 65 more quality years.

There is no single human study I can cite to support my estimates of longevity. We each are different from one another. It is far easier to obtain reliable information about the factors determining the health of guinea pigs or monkeys than of human beings, and I have relied to some extent on the studies made on these and other animal species.

It is my hope that you will find *Look Younger, Live Longer* to contain practical tips, fresh ideas, and most of all, inspiration to encourage your empowerment.

PART I

THE AGING PROCESS

...let your body take advantage
of the wonderful longevity
that Nature originally
designed for it.

THE BIOLOGY OF AGING

W e can turn to the Old Testament to get an idea about the longevity of our species. Many gerontologists ignore Genesis 5:27, which reads, "All the days of Methuselah were nine hundred sixty and nine years and he died," but in the next chapter of Genesis we are informed that "Man's days shall be one hundred and twenty years." This was the age Moses was reported to have reached when he died.

The German writer Goethe completed his masterpiece, *Faust*, at age 83.

These biblical gerontologists were quite accurate. Scientists today estimate the maximum life span of humans to be from 115 to 140 years, with 120 being the most frequently used number.

Pliny the Elder described centenarians in Ancient Rome over 2,000 years ago. A popular actress of that time was one example he cited. Since my office is in Los Angeles and I have several actors and actresses as patients, I can unequivocally state that today's performers share Pliny's interest in passing the century mark.

The Old Testament refers to three score and ten (70) as the average life expectancy of man. Today's biostatisticans tell us that 75 is the average life expectancy in America. The real question is what happens in the gap between 75 and 120 years.

This chapter will answer that query and validate the famous American neurosurgeon Wilder Penfield, who foresaw a day when "more men and women reach life's true goal, fulfilling the cycle set for us, bypassing the plagues, disease and famine."[1]

A Historical Search for the Fountain of Youth

Several thousand years ago the Chinese developed an "anti-aging cocktail" called "Tan." This was made from the toxic metals mercury and gold. Those who sampled this attempt at youthing found themselves in an early grave.

Meditation, nutrition, sports, and even sex were seen by the Taoist religion as the means to prolong life. As we will see this was not far off from the youthing plan presented in part II. In biblical times Middle Eastern societies taught that living to a ripe old age was God's reward for faith and right-living. One's behavior—not an elixir—was the key to longevity, according to these civilizations. When someone attained these goals they were considered models of correct living, and both honor and reverence were bestowed on these long-living citizens. Arabic literature mentioned a Well of Life that would confer youth on those who bathed in its waters. Two thousand years later Ponce de Leon would search for its equivalent in Florida.

During the Middle Ages, Europeans used alchemy to create nostrums they thought would prolong life. This obsession lasted several hundred years. One scholarly work, written in the sixteenth century, explained that aging was the result of the loss of "vital particles" that were exhaled with each breath. The way to stay young, the book suggested, was discovered in the occupant of an ancient Egyptian tomb who had lived an impressive 115 years. According to the inscription on the burial vault, he owed his longevity to "the Breath of Young Women."

---

1   W. Penfield, *The Mystery of the Mind: A Critical Study of Consciousness and the Human Brain* (Princeton: Princeton University Press, 1975).

A description of Shangri-La by James Hilton in his book *Lost Horizon* (publisher, 1930) generated excitement about longevity possibilities. Hilton studied the Supernormals we will discuss in chapter 4 as the model for his book.

Gerovital-H3 was created in the 1950s by Romanian biochemist Ana Aslan. She touted this as an anti-aging drug, but it has failed to demonstrate life-extending characteristics after intensive research spanning 45 years.

L-DOPA, NDGA, SOD, and BHT are examples of purported anti-aging wonder drugs. None of these medications have demonstrated a true solution to the aging problem.

My approach is entirely natural to slow down the aging process (actually reverse it in some cases) and increase our life expectancy by adding 25 to 50 quality years to our existence.

The Effects of Aging

Aging is defined by conventional scientists as the process of growing old and approaching normal death. The process is accompanied by a gradual deterioration in biochemical and physiological functions, such as the activity of enzymes, beginning at about age 35 and continuing at an increasing rate thereafter.

As we grow older these changes have been noted in our body:

- Blood pressure rises by about 15 percent between ages 30 and 65.

- Cholesterol levels rise.

- Blood levels of abnormal proteins increase. Of special significance is the rise in the rheumatoid factor, considered a cause of arthritic joint inflammation.

- By the age of seventy:
    Blood flow to the brain decreases by 20 percent.
    Kidney filtration rate decreases by 50 percent.
    Resting heart output decreases by 30 percent.

Lung volume during exercise decreases by 47 percent.
Oxygen uptake decreases by 60 percent.
Body water content decreases by 15 percent.
Basal metabolic rate decreases by 20 percent.
Brain weight decreases by 40 percent.
Speed of blood equilibrium mechanism decreases by 83 percent.

- The average American man will lose up to 2¾ inches in height between 25 and 70; women will shrink up to 1⅞ inches.

- Hair will lose about one-fifth of its thickness.

- The ear lobe lengthens.

- Aging spots (liver spots) appear.

- The eyes become far-sighted.

- Bags form below the eyes.

- Cheek and jowl skin sags.

- The nose widens and lengthens.

- Lines form around the mouth and eyes.

- Hair becomes gray and balding, mostly in men.

- Muscle coordination and reflexes decline by 25 to 35 percent.

- The skin loses some of its elasticity, especially if there is much exposure to the sun.

From this brief survey you can see how our body's function deteriorates with advancing age. What is omitted from this list is a decline in mental or cognitive function. The National Institute on Aging (NIA) states: "At all ages the majority of people maintain their levels of intellectual competence—or actually improve—as they grow older."[2] *The Handbook for the Biology of Aging* in 1985 averred, "In every age group,

---

2   National Institute on Aging, "With the Passage of Time: The Baltimore Longitudinal Study of Aging." *N.I.H.* Pub. No. 93–3685 (Washington: U.S. Govt. Printing Office, 1993).

even among the oldest, individuals were found whose performance on mental tasks did not decline with age, but was indistinguishable from that of younger adults."[3]

Physicians naturally assumed that since our brains shrank and lost millions of neurons (nerve cells) each year, decreased reasoning ability, memory loss, and impaired intelligence must result. Nerve cells cannot regenerate, and once lost, they are gone forever.

Recent studies have shown that, barring depression, loneliness, lack of outside stimulation, and other forms of psychological distress, over 80 percent of healthy Americans suffer no significant memory loss as they age. Long-term memory actually improves with age!

Younger people do have a slightly better short-term memory. Studies matching 70-year-olds with 20-year-olds demonstrated that the older group could almost match the younger subjects, who were at their prime of mental functioning. Being mentally active can assure that you will retain all facets of intelligence, despite losing over one billion neurons throughout your life.

One medical reason for this retention of intelligence rests in the fact that our dendrites continue to grow throughout our life, up to advanced old age. Dendrites are the parts of our nervous system that function as contact points, allowing the neuron to send signals to its neighbors. By growing new dendrites, a neuron can open new channels of communication in every direction. This may account for the wisdom observed among the elderly.

My own medical training illustrated this principle firsthand. One of my dental school professors was well into his seventies and possessed one of the sharpest minds I had the pleasure of working with during my four years there. We also had a guest lecturer who was in his eighties, and as mentally competent as most people I know who are half his age. The concept of demonstrating a sharp intellect and highly developed memory, as we will see later on, is not unusual with advancing years.

---

3   National Institute on Aging, The *Handbook for the Biology of Aging* (Washington: U.S. Govt. Printing Office, 1985).

Switching On and Off to Life Genetically

All of the cells that make up the human body contain the same package of genetic information that directs what they do, how and when they do it, and how and when they stop doing it. A fertilized human egg (a single cell), containing 46 chromosomes, will convert itself into a multi-trillion-celled adult human being.

These chromosomes are made up of DNA molecules, and these chemically coded spiral lattices contain the entire hereditary future of an individual human. Since there are environmental interactions with these genes, the genes represent only a *potential* of what the individual may become.

The genetic coding of each DNA molecule is copied exactly every time the cell divides. Every cell we have, in fact, contains the entire genetic manual, though any single cell or group of cells uses but a small fraction of this information. After the first few cell divisions of embryonic life, new cells already begin to differentiate; that is, they become more specialized.

RNA (ribonucleic acid) is similar to DNA in coding and structure. Whereas DNA is a double-stranded helix and capable of replicating, RNA is single-stranded and cannot make copies of itself.

The mechanism of the manufacture of protein (the building blocks of life) is as follows: DNA uses enzymes and the assistance of RNA to convert amino acids into proteins. The genetic orders issued by DNA are carried from the nucleus (where both DNA and RNA reside) by enzymes to the cell's cytoplasm. It is here that the very small amino acid molecules are assembled into much larger protein molecules. DNA, RNA and these enzymes are all large molecules. When this assembly line functions properly, the cell is healthy. This process theoretically could go on forever and we would all then be immortal. Aging problems result from a disruption in this protein assembly mechanism.

Certain genes begin to be switched off, or inactivated chemically, very early in embryonic life. Certain proteins (repressors) are made especially for this purpose. These very same genes are later turned on by derepressor proteins, who act to deactivate the repressors. During embryonic and fetal development, genes are constantly being switched on and off, so that cells know when to divide and when to stop dividing.

A series of proteins called *chromatin* reside alongside the DNA in the nucleus. These nuclear proteins are reported to be responsible for turning the genes on and off. Some genes, it is believed, may turn on only once in the cell's lifetime, providing the blueprint needed for one specific chemical product, then turn off again forever. The exact "start" and "stop" signals for some genes are beginning to be known. This data will prove invaluable in unlocking nature's secrets regarding the process of aging.

Cells are constantly dying and being replaced during the entire pre-natal period. In fact, more cells die before birth than die at death! In an article in *Science*, Joan Whitten points out the importance of cell death to the proper formation of fingers, toes, arms, and legs. By chemically interfering with cell death during a critical point in the in utero for-mation of the digits of lab animals, these digits grew together in a webbed fashion rather than with spaces between them as nature had intended. Whitten had saved the lives of the cells that were pro-grammed to die, but, in so doing, she had crippled the animal! Such life-saving mistakes occur during human embryonic development and result in birth defects.

Whitten observed two different forms of programmed cell death. "In the vertebrate limb the death clocks function on time even when the tissue is transferred to a host of different age," which she takes as strong proof that "the timing of the vertebrate death clock is independent of external factors."[4]

Pathologist J. N. Webb verified Whitten's conclusions and in *Nature* wrote that such cell death "takes place in a highly predictable manner

---

4   J. Whitten, "Cell Death During Early Morphogenesis: Parallels between Insect Limb and Vertebrae Limb Development" (*Science*, March 28, 1969).

and all the evidence points to it being genetically controlled."[5] Webb believes that the programmed death of these cells "must…serve a function which is probably crucial to the subsequent healthy development and growth of that tissue." The failure of the death switches to operate on schedule may result in their switching on at a later time of life. This could cause a disease such as muscular dystrophy. In that case, Webb believes, the disease could be looked upon "as a normal process, but one occurring at the wrong time in the individual's life span—or else one which has not been repressed."

In biology, growth is the transformation of the developing being from one stage to the next and so on. There is no scientific reason that this rate of cell destruction at the beginning of life can't be lowered as we age. Furthermore, a spurt of acceleration of cells toward the end of our life cycle is not out of the question. For example, when the silkworm turns into a moth, enormous quantities of cells must die and new ones be created to bring about the birth of a being that bears no resemblance to the one from which it emerged.

The existence of cells that specifically regulate aging has been proposed by Holger P. von Hahn of the Institute of Experimental Gerontology in Basel, Switzerland. That there are as many as 70 genes involved in aging has been suggested by George M. Martin of the University of Washington School of Medicine in Seattle. USC's Bernard Strehler, Florida's Leonard Hayflick, UCLA's Roy Walford and NIA's Richard G. Cutler feel that only a few regulatory genes are involved in the "clock of aging." They suspect a clustered "supergene" may be the key.

This genetic switching on and off is important, not just for cell division, but for its cessation. *Mitotic* cells continue to divide throughout life, whereas resting or *postmitotic* cells cease this replication once the organism attains full growth. Still other cells are in between those two classes and do not ordinarily divide, but can begin doing so again when circumstances demand it. Liver cells serve as a good example of this

---

5 J. N. Webb, "Muscular Dystrophy and Muscle Cell Death in Normal Foetal Development" (*Nature,* November 15, 1974).

in-between category. They appear to be postmitotic, but if a piece of the liver is cut away or damaged, the division switches are somehow turned on again in response to the challenge, and they spring into action until the missing piece is regenerated, at which point they turn off again.

Among the cells that are mitotic are those that line the gastrointestinal tract, skin cells, red and white blood cells and the lymphocytes of our immune system. Postmitotic cell examples are cells of the nerves and muscles. If we can turn on heart cells, we can increase the survival rate of victims of heart attacks by regenerating heart muscle cells. The same principle applies to stroke victims where brain cells might be regenerated or "turned on."

Some estimates state that as many as 100,000 brain cells die each day after the age of 35, under normal aging biology. Even with the billions of brain cells we initially have, this is not a negligible loss.

The Operon Theory

The Nobel Prize team of Francois Jacob and Jacques Moned, at the Pasteur Institute in Paris, developed the "operon theory." This role of nucleoproteins (chromosomes being composed of DNA and associated proteins called chromatin described earlier) generated our first real insights into the actual mechanism of genetic on/off switching. The knowledge acquired up to the mid-1970s was carefully spelled out in a 1975 *Scientific American* article by Gary S. Stein and Janet Swinehart Stein of the University of Florida, in collaboration with Lewis J. Klinesmith of the University of Michigan. Today this understanding of nucleoproteins holds up quite well.

Histones

Holger von Hahn, Alfred E. Mirsky and Vincent G. Allfry of the Rockefeller University, James Bonner, and others have identified *histones* as the chief repressor proteins. These "off" switches monitor the parts of the DNA containing the information designed to be off-limits for the messenger-RNA molecules delegated the role of transcribing the genetic data.

The manufacture of messenger-RNA molecules also ceases when that information is repressed. This is an added measure to ensure that nothing will reactivate a switched-off gene. It is *non-histone* nucleoproteins that assist the histones in turning on a gene again. The enzymes in the nucleus that are responsible for replication, repair and other activities in the cells are comprised of these non-histone nucleoproteins.

Whereas the quantity of histones remains stable (just enough to repress the genetic information on all of the DNA molecules in a particular chromosome), the non-histones vary considerably in their presence at any given time—often depending on the number of genes that are turned on or off and the quantity of messenger-RNA molecules that are on hand.

In a series of experiments carried out by F. Marott Sinex and his associates at the Boston University School of Medicine, three consistent sets of results were noted with respect to aging.

- The number of derepressors (non-histones) goes down.

- The making of chromatin RNA decreases.

- The number of repressors (histones) rises.[6]

It is clear that this causes more genes to be turned off as the cell ages.

We know that DNA is the set of genetic instructions contained in each of our cells. Does this make DNA the library or the librarian? One possibility is that the true intelligence in the regulation of our gene rests in certain non-histone proteins. These may use the passive DNA as a blueprint to be activated only at the time and to the extent that such use is appropriate. Regulator genes do exist, including repressor genes, along with genes that direct the manufacture of the repressor proteins.

6   F. Marott Sinex, "Genetic Mechanisms of Aging" (*Journal of Gerontology,* July 1966).

There is no current answer to the genetic question, "which came first, the Histone (chicken) or the DNA (egg)?"

Stein and Kleinsmith predicted in their 1975 *Scientific American* article, "It may not be long before proteins that regulate the expression of specific genes are isolated, introducing the possibility of a certain kind of genetic engineering: the proteins might be inserted into cells in order to modify abnormalities in gene transcription associated with development, differentiation and a broad spectrum of diseases, including cancer. Such a capability might revolutionize man's ability to deal with some profoundly destructive disorders."[7]

Chapter 6 presents various theories on aging. I believe that any theory of cellular aging must encompass both mitotic and postmitotic cells, as well as those in-between categories, in all their diversity of types. We would expect that if the same packet of DNA can program the cells to develop so differently, and to live such different existences, it can surely program them to age and die differently as well.

Our knowledge of genes and the proteins that turn them on and off could empower us once and for all to put an end to the most destructive disorder of all time—old age itself.

---

7   J. Stein and L. J. Kleinsmith, "Chromosomal Proteins and Gene Regulation" (*Scientific American*, February 1975).

OUR IMMUNE SYSTEM

Without a properly functioning immune system, we wouldn't live past birth. The secret of looking younger and living a longer and more fulfilled life lies in keeping this immune system operating as efficiently and effectively as possible. Our immune system, however, is one of the first bodily systems to deteriorate with advancing age.

At 89, Albert Schweitzer was still operating a hospital in Africa.

- Most classic "diseases of aging," such as heart disease, arthritis, cancer, and pneumonia, occur only after our immune system begins to lose its potency.

- Scientists consider that the immune system is controlled by the same genes that guide the aging process.

- The immune system begins to attack itself (autoimmune diseases such as arthritis) upon aging.

- When the aging immune system loses its efficiency in cleansing the body of defective and dead normal cells, this build-up of cellular garbage facilitates the aging of other organs.

Components of the Immune System

Two groups of cells comprise our immune system. White blood cells (*leukocytes*) are examples of this first group. The main activity of these *phagocytes* (scavenger cells) is to engulf and eat foreign invaders to the body.

Lymphocytes make up the second group of cells making up our immune system. This is a far more important group, having the capability to recognize and respond to individual enemies to the body. T-cells and B-cells are lymphocytes. These scavengers are made in the lymph glands and function in lymphs (a suspension of the cells in a clear yellowish fluid resembling blood plasma) through the lymphatic vessels to the bloodstream. The lymphocytes seem to be the most important of the phagocytic cells in the battles against cancer and other diseases. A malignant tumor is often observed to be infiltrated with lymphocytes, and a high degree of lymphocyte infiltration is now accepted as a reliable indicator of a favorable outcome of the disease.

B-cells function as foot soldiers in the immune system army. They produce substances called antibodies (immunoglobins) that stimulate a sequence of other chemical reactions. The result of this biochemistry is the destruction of a specific invader, without harming the body itself.

A more interesting characteristic of a B-cell is its ability to "remember" an invading cell. Should that invader return, the B-cell quickly dispenses its antibodies and the invading cell now meets a quicker death, as compared to its predecessor. This, for example, accounts for our permanent immunity to childhood diseases, once we have had the illness.

Vaccines contain weakened or dead strains of dangerous viruses or bacteria. By assembling this false attack, our B-cells mobilize and are now prepared to fight off a real attack, such as cold viruses during the influenza season.

Continuing with our army analogy, the T-cells represent the

sergeants and lieutenants. They direct the fighting and participate in it themselves. Various subgroups of T-cells work together to control the immune army through a complex system of chemical commands. T-cells help stimulate the immune system when danger is imminent and slow down the immune response when it gets too strong. Whereas B-cells conduct their fighting from a distance, T-cells combat at close range. These T-cells are our prime defense against cancer cells.

More recently discovered components of the immune system are the *interferons.* These agents are produced by cells infected by a virus. Some scientists feel that malignant cells may manufacture this substance. In any event, interferons are proteins that kill viruses. They assist other cells in the body to resist infection. There is some evidence that interferons help in the effort by the human body to control a developing cold or other infection or cancer. We make about twenty different kinds of interferon molecules, each kind engaging in somewhat different activities in different cells in the body. This is important because most drugs are ineffective against cancer and other viral infections (AIDS, for example).

Prostaglandins are small molecules that play an important role in our immune system. These lipids (fats) function as hormones and aid in the regulation of the heartbeat and the responses of the immune system. Whenever any tissue is disturbed or damaged it releases prostaglandins. The prostaglandins are involved with other substances in producing inflammation of the tissues—redness, swelling, pain, tenderness, and heat—resulting from increased flow of blood and the movement of leukocytes and other cells and substances to the region in response to the hormones.

The master gland of the immune system is the thymus. It functions as a command center for T-cells and as an officer's training school. Immature white blood cells, the raw recruits, travel from the bone marrow to the thymus to be turned into mature, functioning T-cells. The thymus also makes hormones that circulate throughout the body and help T- and B-cells interact effectively.

While each component of the immune system is important on its own, no single part can work effectively without the others helping out. We still have much to learn about our immune system.

The Effects of Normal Aging on the Immune System

Our immune system is one of the first to be compromised by normal aging. The master gland of the immune system, our thymus is a pink, flat, two-lobed gland located under the sternum. It weighs about 1½ ounces when we are about eleven years old, but begins to shrink quickly with the onset of puberty. When we turn 40 it is only 10 to 15 percent of the size it was at age 11. One obvious result of this shrinkage is a decline in the production of hormones that organize and direct the B-cells and T-cells. The thymus also becomes less effective in converting immature white blood cells into fully functioning T-cells, and as those all-important T-cells are less able to do their job, the whole immune army is thrown out of step. Because the thymus deteriorates early, the immune system's power peaks in adolescence and goes downhill from there.

This deterioration is more a qualitative than a quantitative one. The number of white blood cells we possess at age 80 is about the same as when we were 20 years old, but these senile white blood cells are less effective in receiving and transmitting commands. They may also experience difficulty in reaching their proper destination.

Now the entire immune system is compromised. B- and T-cells no longer coordinate their actions to destroy and remove invading organisms. This results in older people becoming more susceptible to infection. An increase in the rates of influenza, pneumonia, tuberculosis, and other diseases in the elderly bear this out.

Cancer incidences are of particular concern to us today. Scientists assume that our body produces cancer cells at a fairly consistent rate throughout life. Younger immune systems (mostly through T-cells) are more efficient in identifying and killing these malignant cells before they multiply and spread throughout the body. Older immune systems simply allow more of these cancer cells to "get by the goalie."

Autoimmune Disease

The one antibody that does seem to strengthen as we age is an autoimmune type. This is most undesirable, since its presence causes our body to literally attack itself.

B-cells begin producing autoantibodies targeted to the lining of our blood vessels, nerves, and other normal cells in response to the errors made by our aging immune system. Our own cells now become labeled as the enemy by the B-cells. Autoantibodies can be found in the blood of nearly every older American, and researchers suspect they play a part in conditions ranging from heart disease and arthritis to neurological ailments.

The T-cells actually cause this collapse of the normally highly efficient immune system. By loosening the T-cells' control over the B-cells, the B-cells are allowed to produce increasing quantities of autoantibodies. Researchers have found that people with higher concentrations of autoantibodies in their blood tend to run increased risks of cancer and heart disease, and have generally shorter life spans.

We really don't know exactly why the T-cells degenerate in function or why the thymus shrinks. I suspect it is due to a decrease in the adrenal androgen DHEA, which is discussed in chapter 5. The following table lists diseases that result from the production of autoantibodies.

DISEASE	PART OF BODY ATTACKED
Rheumatoid arthritis	Joint linings
Graves disease	Thyroid gland
Multiple sclerosis	Nerve fibers
Diabetes	Pancreas cells
Hepatitis	Liver

The combination of incompetent T- and B-cells, elevated autoantibody levels, and a shrinking thymus adds up to a weaker immune system with advancing years. Still, our immune system serves us quite well throughout our life. Phagocytes don't appear to lose any of their power with age. Although our ability to fight off a new infection declines with age, our immune memory response remains unimpaired throughout life. That allows our body to continue to fight off most infections, especially those we've been exposed to before.

Middle age and beyond does not signal the likelihood of cancer or a significant increase in other infections and diseases. This is the basis of my thesis. We can keep this beautifully designed system functioning the way nature intended and eliminate our vulnerability to "diseases of aging." It is possible to significantly increase our longevity, while maintaining a high quality of life.

The "Exquisite Relationship"

The interaction between the conscious mind, the subconscious, the physical brain, the endocrine system (hormones) and the immune system has been referred to as the "exquisite relationship." We will discuss the relationship in detail in chapter 7, when I develop the effects of consciousness on aging.

Carl Simonton, a radiation oncologist, and Stephanie Matthews-Simonton, a psychotherapist, combined visual imagery techniques with hypnosis to fight cancer nearly 30 years ago.[1] Their approach involves having the cancer patient first relax, then visualizing his or her immune system's white blood cells attacking and destroying "weak, confused" cancer cells in their body like "strong, powerful" sharks attacking meat. Patients were also encouraged to develop other images that follow the same theme.

---

1   O. C. Simonton, S. Matthews-Simonton, and J. L. Creighton, *Getting Well Again* (Los Angeles: Tarcher-St. Martin's Press, 1978).

The Simontons clinically tested this procedure with 159 selected patients diagnosed with medically incurable cancer and given one year to live. Their results were remarkable. Sixty-three of the original 159 patients were alive two years after their diagnosis; recall that this was one year longer than their original prognosis. Even more interesting, of those sixty-three patients who had practiced the visualization/relaxation procedure and were alive two years later, 22.2 percent showed no evidence of cancer, 19.1 percent demonstrated tumor regression, while 27.1 percent of these patients had stabilized. The Simontons attempted to account for these findings by postulating that the visualization/relaxation procedure resulted in an enhancement of the patient's immune system.

According to Campbell and Stanley,[2] the work of the Simontons suggests two interesting hypotheses. One, it should be possible to raise immune functioning in the laboratory under controlled conditions. Second, hypnotizability may be related to one's ability to produce such alterations. This study thus concluded that hypnosis and visualization may result in increased immune function for certain individuals.

A number of studies have suggested that hypnosis may result in alterations of immune functions. For example, allergic reactions can be inhibited with hypnosis and suggestion. Lymphocyte function can also be increased with hypnosis and visualization.

The work of Kiecolt-Glaser,[3] for instance, demonstrated an increase in T-cell levels in the blood as a result of these hypnotic exercises.

In summary, this exquisite relationship has shown us that the mind can greatly aid our immune system. Here is a brief list of observations made by myself and my colleagues:

- Relaxation techniques designed to ease stress also appear capable of boosting the immune response.

---

2   D. T. Campbell and J. C. Stanley, *Experimental and Quasi-Experimental Designs for Research* (Chicago: Rand McNally, 1973).

3   J. K. Kiecolt-Glaser, and others, "Psychosocial Enhancement of Immuncompetence in a Geriatric Population," *Health Psychology* 4 (1985): 25-41.

- Physicians are testing the effects of "hope-enhancing exercises" and visualization techniques, as well as behavior and attitude, on patients with severe diseases.

- Researchers are taking a new look at the effects of placebos— inactive substances that sometimes result in miraculous cures if the patient believes they're effective.

- The effect of stress on the immune system appears to depend on how much control the subjects feel they have over their situation. Feelings of helplessness, depression and anxiety worsen the immune-system decline.

Successful application of these techniques to cases of cancer and AIDS, as well as several other diseases, are presented in my book, *Soul Healing* (Llewellyn Publications, 1996).

The Disease Bank

Every insult to the body, every illness, every stress increases the physiological age of a person and decreases his or her life expectancy. The amounts by which life expectancy is decreased due to episodes of illness have been reported by Dr. Hardin Jones of the Donner Laboratory of Medical Physics of the University of California in Berkeley.[4] He points out that there is evidence that aging results from damage to the bodily functions. Among these damaging episodes are illnesses; each illness leaves the body with decreased ability to function in an optimum way. One disease experience tends to lead to another and to decrease life expectancy. This effect could be illustrated by saying that each person is born with a certain amount of vitality, that some vitality is used up by each episode of illness or other causes of stress, and that death comes when the quota of vitality has been exhausted. It is equivalent to over-drawing on your bank account.

---

4 H. B. Jones, *Sensual Drugs: Deprivation and Rehabilitation of the Mind* (Boston: Cambridge University Press, 1976).

Jones concludes that the way to avoid disease is by not having earlier diseases: "…we may be able to achieve an even greater preservation of physiologic health by the elimination of our more trivial diseases; the successful removal of such 'benign' diseases as the common cold, chicken pox, measles, etc., may be more effective in lessening the disease tendency of later life than anything else we may attempt to do."[5]

By keeping our immune system strong we can decrease the amount and duration of these and other illnesses. Our immune system bank can expand with its compound interest, and we can draw on this account to live longer and healthier.

---

5   H. B. Jones, op. cit.

3

NATURE PLANNED FOR US TO LIVE TO 120 OR OLDER

Would it surprise you to know that our life span has not increased significantly in the past 6,000 years? The life span of humans was 70 to 100 years in Greece 2,500 years ago, almost exactly what it is today. However, the ancient Greeks had a life expectancy of only 22 years.

At 88 Konrad Adenauer was Chancellor of Germany.

Bodily functions lose approximately one percent of their original capacity each year from the age of 30, according to gerontologist Dr. Nathan Schock.[1] Mathematically this computes out to a natural life span of at least 120 years for humans.

Mental decline is not supposed to occur with advancing age. Dr. Richard L. Sprott of the Jackson Laboratory at Bar Harbor, Maine, has demonstrated that our I.Q. remains constant throughout our life.[2] It does not matter how long we live, the human intelligence quotient remains the same. Other studies have since shown that very few mental functions decline with age. Senility is not automatic as we grow older. This disease is brought on by specific medical problems, and can be successfully treated if diagnosed early enough.

---

1 N. Shock, R. C. Greulich, et al, *Normal Human Aging* (Washington: U.S. Government Printing Office, 1984).
2 R. L. Sprott, *Age, Learning Ability and Intelligence* (New York: Van Nostrand Reinhold, 1980).

A life expectancy of 120 years is quite possible (if not conservative). What has prevented us from achieving this level (other than the 15 percent who are supernormals) are psychological and consciousness blocks. The life extension techniques presented in Part II will unquestionably work. The question is when. The sooner you begin their implementation, the faster the techniques will become a part of your reality.

In chapter 1, I described the mechanism of protein manufacture by our cells (pp. 8–10). A shortened life is due to something going wrong with this protein assembly line. The incorporation of errors in this series of processes results in miscopying the genetic information in succeeding generations of DNA and RNA. The compounding of these errors has a deleterious effect on our immune system and makes us vulnerable to the diseases of aging.

Controlling all of our DNA might not result in complete immortality, but it certainly would increase the quantity and quality of both our life span and life expectancy by a considerable amount. In part II we will discuss how this can be accomplished by completely natural approaches.

Aging Myths

Dr. Robert N. Butler, former director of the NIA, coined the term *ageism.* "Ageism is the stereotyping, the prejudices, the discrimination that surrounds old age," he says. "All of which is really based on the underlying personal dread we have about growing old."[3]

No one is more insulted and offended by ageism than Dr. Butler. He points specifically to the common use of such terms as decrepit, dependent, doddering, ineffectual, and confused when describing older people—and his book, *Why Survive? Being Old in America,* won a Pulitzer Prize.

---

3 Robert Butler, *Why Survive? Being Old in America* (New York: Harper & Row, 1975).

Myth # 1 — Old People Become Senile

It is true that we are constantly losing brain cells (100,000 daily is the accepted range) and that they cannot be replaced (postmitotic). We are born with 100 billion brain cells, and certain parts of our brain don't experience a cell loss no matter how old we become.

I have already pointed out that I.Q. and cognitive functions do not decline with age. Senility isn't even a medical disorder—it is psychological at best. What many people have is *gerontophobia*—the fear of old age. As the English satirist Jonathan Swift stated, "Every man desires to live long, but no man would be old."

In the absence of real disease or brain damage, chances are that intellectual decline is minor and not progressive. It usually does not keep getting worse. Investigator Barry Riesberg of New York University has found that most of these worries are groundless; that, in fact, the worriers are the ones who usually don't have to worry—the elderly person who really has a mental problem probably isn't aware of it.[4]

Myth # 2 — Older People Are No Longer Productive

The list of productive people in their seventies, eighties and beyond is rather long. One of the greatest tragedies of retirement is the waste of talent it can represent. Some of our most impressive accomplishments came from people who were over 65...over 75...over 100.

Here is a list of some famous people who nicely illustrate the principle of youthing and longevity:

- Thomas Edison was in his eighties when he invented the dictaphone and the duplicating machine. He had already invented the light bulb and the phonograph.

- At 89 Albert Schweitzer was running a hospital in Africa.

- Grandma Moses was an active artist at 100.

- Pablo Picasso was still painting at 92.

---

4 Barry Riesberg, *Brain Failure: An Introduction to Current Concepts of Senility* (New York: The Free Press, 1981).

- Leo Tolstoy wrote *I Cannot Be Silent* at 82.

- Michelangelo, who painted the ceiling of the Sistine Chapel, was still painting at 88.

- Armand Hammer, in his 90s, ran a multibillion-dollar empire.

- At 88 Konrad Adenauer was Chancellor of Germany.

- At 89 Mary Baker Eddy was directing the Christian Science Church.

- W. Somerset Maugham wrote *Points of View* at 84.

- Sophocles wrote *Oedipus at Colonus* at age 92.

- At 91 Eamon de Valera served as President of Ireland.

- Irving Berlin, at age 101, continued to compose music.

- Winston Churchill wrote *A History of the English-Speaking Peoples* at 82.

- Also, George Bernard Shaw continued to write witty plays when he was in his late eighties. Coco Chanel, the distinguished leader of Parisian fashion, engineered a success comeback (after retiring at age 55) at the age of 71. Benjamin Franklin was 81 when he mediated the compromise that led to the adoption of the U.S. Constitution. George Burns became a dramatic actor and starred in *The Sunshine Boys* at 79. He continued his movie career and lived to be 100!

Myth # 3 — Older People Are Always Ill

Dr. Richard Butler in his book, *Why Survive? Being Old in America,* states quite clearly that only 5 percent of people over 65 are in nursing homes. He points out that the majority of them are able to care for themselves. Gerontologist Alex Comfort, M.D., cites statistics in his book, *A Good Age,* that people over 65 have only about half as many acute illnesses per year as do people of all ages.

Studies conducted by the Corporate Committee for Retirement Planning make it clear that older employees have no more absences and on-the-job accidents than younger ones. Ninety-seven percent of the personnel directors queried in this survey stated that older workers have better attendance records than do their younger counterparts. Over half of these personnel directors affirmed the fact that older workers have fewer on-the-job accidents than younger ones.

Myth # 4 — Sex Is Either Impossible or Unenjoyable after 60

If your sexual drive is strong and sexual activity vigorous in your middle years, you are likely to have a comparatively vigorous sex life well into your seventies. A weak sex drive at midlife is unlikely to improve in your golden years.

William H. Masters and Virginia E. Johnson, of the internationally respected Masters and Johnson clinic in St. Louis, state that healthy men and women can enjoy an active sex life well into their eighties. A satisfying sex life can and should continue indefinitely if sexual confidence is not destroyed by unrealistic expectations.

Myth # 5 — Old People Are Lonely and Poor

Studies show that 28 percent of all discretionary money is held by older consumers. Most Americans over 65 own their own homes. The per capita household income of domiciles headed by someone over 65 is only $500.00 lower than the rest of the population.

Luxury cruises are predominantly taken by people over 55. These older Americans make up a special, affluent leisure class. More than half of older citizens see or speak with their families almost every day. Over sixty percent of these older people see or talk to friends nearly every day.

Myth # 6 — Older People Are Sedentary

There is no medical reason that older people can't be active. In fact, many are. Fred Knoller was named by *50 Plus* magazine as one of the top athletes of 1981. He was 86 at the time and a tournament bicyclist.

Playing golf, hunting, fishing, swimming, backpacking, jogging, canoeing, or playing tennis and racquetball are regularly practiced by older people all over the world.

Myth # 7 — Creativity Disappears in Old Age

At the age of 78 Benjamin Franklin invented bifocal glasses. Louise Nevelson created a spectacular new exhibit of sculpting at age 78. The feature film director Cecil B. De Mille was 71 when he directed and produced the Academy Award-winning film, *The Greatest Show on Earth.*

Best-selling authors Irving Stone, Taylor Caldwell, and Harold Robbins were productive very late in life. The German writer Goethe completed his masterpiece, *Faust,* when he was 83. Agatha Christie wrote murder mystery novels until she was 84. Frank Lloyd Wright designed the Guggenheim Museum in New York City when he was 76 years old. The list goes on and on (see Myth 2).

Gay Luce, a psychologist who has studied older people, wrote, "As people grow older, they become more intuitive, sensitive and psychic. This is one of the reasons why older people are often more religious. It's also why they can be more creative."[5]

Old Age as a Curable Disease

The death rate increases with age, in consequence of the aging process, but death may be caused at any age by illness, accident, suicide, or murder. Accidents cause about 4.5 percent of all deaths in the United States, suicide about 1.4 percent, homicide about 1.0 percent, and illness about 93 percent. The mortality (death rate) from illness is a measure of the change in health caused by aging.

"Aging and death do seem to be what nature has planned for us," says Bernard L. Strehler, of the University of California. "But what

---

5   Gay Luce, *Your Second Life* (New York: Delacorte Press, 1979).

if we have other plans?"[6] Strehler makes it plain that he, for one, has other plans. He characterizes death as a kind of Moby Dick, a tough, re-morseless leviathan—never before conquered, *but still conquerable.*

Strehler also avers, "Death may be in accord with nature's plan so far. But there is no absolute principle in nature which dictates that individual living things cannot live for indefinitely long periods of time in optimum health."[7] One of gerontology's unabashed aims, then, is this: to cure or prevent the disease we now call old age, or senescence. Its other major aim—to extend the human life span.

In order to cure old age, biomedical science must overcome the Josh Billings Syndrome. Billings once stated, "The trouble with people is not that they don't know, but that they know so much that ain't so."[8] Some very authoritative experts have a tendency to let what they think they know interfere with what they might learn. Arthur C. Clarke once commented on his "law" concerning experts: whenever an expert insists that a problem is impossible to solve, he is certainly premature and almost certainly mistaken. I refer to this as professional ego.

This narrow-minded approach to science prevents inspection of certain hypotheses. Current accepted notions do not always stand the test of time. Weighing future possibilities on the basis of present technique, assumptions, and knowledge is not a successful formula for progress in any field.

As I stated before, the main problem with postponing aging is with DNA duplication. Aging is accompanied by the slowing down of the physiological and biochemical processes that go on in the body, by decreasing strength, and by increasing incidence of illness and probability of death. The molecules of deoxyribonucleic acid (DNA) that control the synthesis of enzymes and other proteins undergo changes (somatic mutations) that lead to decreased production of these important

---

6   Bernard L. Strehler, *Time, Cells and Aging* (New York: Academic Press, 1977).
7   Ibid.
8   D. Kesterson, *Josh Billings* (New York: Twayne, 1973).

substances or to changes in the molecules that decrease their activity. These changes in enzymes throughout the body are compounded by poor nutrition resulting from poor appetite and decreased activity of the digestive enzymes. The increase in the number of cells containing chromosomal abnormality contributes to these effects.

Most people assume that physicians are the best source for helping us prolong life, but few doctors have high cure rates for unhappy lives. In fact, your visit may result in the initiation of a series of potentially dangerous medical tests and treatments.

Some researchers believe the body ages not from overuse but from disuse. "The body," writes Stanford researcher James F. Fries in the *New England Journal of Medicine*, "is now felt to rust out rather than wear out."[9] We can do something about disuse, and that means a great deal of the aging process is within our control. Our state of mind and lifestyle can make a difference in extending our lives. The earlier we concern ourselves, the better our chances of lessening or postponing many of the effects of aging, for not all the changes we think of as inevitable actually are. Most digestive problems are not a consequence of aging. Neither is hardening of the arteries, dental disease, loss of muscle tone or middle-age spread. We don't automatically lose flexibility, endurance and stamina because we grow older. Our memory doesn't automatically worsen; our sex drive doesn't automatically fade.

Most of the alleged diseases of aging are really nothing but the cumulative effects of bad habits exhibited by some people during the late twentieth century, such as watching too much television and lack of exercise, etc. Researchers say inactivity accounts for about half of our functional decline between ages 30 and 70. Scientists say the typical American's high-fat, low-fiber diet is a major cause of heart disease and many digestive disorders. Lack of exercise weakens our muscles— including the most important one, the heart—and contributes to problems ranging from obesity to joint disorders. Smoking, best known for

9   J. F. Fries, *Living Well: Taking Care of Your Health in the Middle and Later Years* (Reading, Mass.: Addison-Wesley Pub. Co., 1994).

its horrific effects on the lungs, also contributes to hardening of the arteries and wrinkled facial skin. Stress can age us inside and out, contributing to both the serious business of heart attacks and the frivolous concern of graying hair.

On the other hand, studies show that relaxation techniques can help keep blood pressure down and facilitate our immune system, as I described earlier. Regular, vigorous exercise can keep our weight down, muscles toned, and heart young. In short, what we *do* makes a difference. We can age well. The key is understanding how we age, and what we can do now to slow the process.

4

THE OVER-100 CLUB

What do the Andean village of Vilcabamba in Ecuador, Abkhazia in the Georgian part of Russia, and the land of Hunza in the Karakoram Range in Pakistan-controlled Kashmir have in common? They are the home of some of the oldest people in the world.

Irving Berlin, at age 101, was still composing music.

People here are believed to remain vigorous and live much longer than those in most industrialized societies. These remote and mountainous regions have been studied by gerontologists for many years.

Physician and Harvard Professor Alexander Leaf traveled to these three regions on a grant from the National Geographic Society in the early 1970s and wrote a rather famous article that appeared in the January 1973 issue of *National Geographic*. He also authored a book, *Youth in Age*, on his studies.[1]

One of the most interesting people he interviewed was in the village of Kutol, in the Caucasus Mountains in Georgia, Russia. Khfaf Lasuria was a short, white-haired woman who claimed to be at least 130 years old. She had worked on a local collective farm as a tea leaf picker since she was 100. She finally retired in 1970.

---

1 Alexander Leaf, "Where Life Begins at 100," *National Geographic* (January 1973).

Khfaf Lasura drank vodka before breakfast and smoked a pack of cigarettes daily. Although there was no baptismal record for Khfaf, Dr. Leaf estimated her age as between 131 and 141.

The Georgian diet consisted of about 1800 calories a day, 600 calories less than recommended by the U.S. National Academy of Sciences for men over 55. Russian studies claimed that the plasma cholesterol level of these centenarians averaged less than half the accepted normal amount for Americans aged 50 to 60.

Dr. Leaf noted an occasional overweight Georgian, but the elderly in Vilcabamba and Hunza were generally quite slim. There were no signs of malnutrition. There was a striking similarity between the diets of Hunza and Vilcabamba, in that they both were significantly lower in calories than those recommended by the U.S. government.

The Mir (ruler) of Hunza could, from personal knowledge of his state's history, verify ages, but it was the fitness of these elderly people that most impressed Dr. Leaf. In all three cultures, regular physical activity was incorporated into their lifestyles.

Being independent and free to participate in activities they wanted to do and enjoyed, along with the maintenance of a placid state of mind free from emotional strain and worry, were emphasized by these centenarians.

Diet cannot be ignored as a factor when comparing these three cultures to the United States. By the time the typical American reaches 65, nearly half of their body weight is fat—double what it was in their twenties. This occurs because our bodies lose muscle mass and replace it with fat.

To be journalistically fair I must report that there were some problems with the accuracy of the age of some of the Abkhasians. Khfaf Lazuria died in 1975 at the alleged age of 140, but many inconsistencies about her stories to journalists surfaced.

She freely changed her age and the number of husbands she claimed to have had. Every visitor was told something different. No records could be found since over 90 percent of the local churches (the only place these records would be maintained) had been destroyed by Stalin.

You can imagine the advantage politically for the then Soviet government to use centenarian propaganda as a testimonial to the Communist lifestyle. Some feel this was a deliberate hoax by the Soviets for this very purpose.

My feeling is that there may very well have been some fudging by the Soviets. Maybe Khfaf Lazuria wasn't 140. However, there were definitely centenarians in Abkhasia, a lot of them. Nobody doubts that these 100-year-old-plus people occupied villages in Vilcabamba in Ecuador and Hunza in Pakistan.

Previous studies corroborated Leaf's work. Flanders Dunbar, a professor of medicine at Columbia University, in 1955 reported on a study of centenarians. The most notable trait Dr. Dunbar observed among these people was psychological adaptability in the face of stress. As part of her research, Dunbar listed six traits that were shared by "precentenarians," people who have the best chance of living to be 100:

- The capacity to integrate new things into one's existence.

- Responding creatively to change. More than any other, this trait made precentenarians stand out from ordinary people.

- Wanting to stay alive.

- Freedom from anxiety.

- The continued ability to create and invent.

- High levels of adaptive energy.[2]

The mid-life period of 45 to 65 is the most difficult period for us to survive in our quest for a longer life. It is during this time that alcoholism, elevated cholesterol, poor genes, smoking, and other negative factors take their highest toll.

---

2   Flanders Dunbar, *Mind and Body Psychosomatic Medicine* (New York: Random House, 1955).

Of all the factors affecting longevity, frugal eating criteria has received most of the attention of individuals trying to extend their life span. Luigi Cornaro, a fifteenth-century Venetian nobleman who lived an unhealthy lifestyle in his youth, vowed to make amends and was determined to reach 100 years of age.

Cornaro was good to his word. He ate sparingly, abstained from drinking, and generally followed the ancient Greek and Roman notions of a frugal diet being the key to longevity. He lived to the age of 103 and remained in possession of his mental and physical faculties until the very end of his life. The average Venetian of Cornaro's day lived to be only 35!

NIA researcher Richard Greulich coined the term "supernormals" to describe these people. He noted the following common traits among these individuals:

- Their attitudes toward leisure activities, security, health, and friendships are the same as those of younger people.

- They have strong feelings about being useful.

- They tend to be well-educated or come from high-level, high-responsibility jobs.

- They tend to be extroverted and remain socially active.

Greulich noted an empowerment characteristic of these supernormals. They started out mentally active, often attaining a high level of formal education, and often taking on high-powered jobs. After retirement, they stay intellectually active and involved. A job with responsibility and rewards gives supernormals a feeling of usefulness, and working part-time, whether volunteer or paid, keeps that feeling alive, even though this job may not be as challenging as their previous career.[3]

Even under the most stressful tests—on stationary bicycles in the lab, for instance, where the subjects "rode" without letup as hard as they

---

3   R. Greulich, N. Shock, et al, *Normal Human Aging*.

could until totally exhausted—the supernormals maintained essentially the same cardiac output as other participants who were in their twenties and thirties. There was an important difference in how the bodies of the older people did the job, however: the heart rate did not increase nearly so much as that of the younger subjects, but the stroke volume—the amount of blood pumped with each heartbeat—increased to compensate for the slower rate.

DHEA — NATURE'S FOUNTAIN OF YOUTH

One of the strangest hormones to be associated with aging is dehydroepiandrosterone (DHEA), which is produced by the adrenal glands and gonads. Though it is the most abundant steroid hormone circulating in our bloodstream, until recently endocrinologists were reluctant even to classify it as a hormone; it had no known function, and it simply didn't act the way hormones are supposed to.

At age 92, Sophocles wrote *Oedipus at Colonus.*

Scientists observed back in the 1950s that DHEA production reaches its peak at the age of about twenty-five years and declines steadily thereafter, going down virtually in a straight line with age. No other steroid hormone behaves this way. Research by Claude Migeon at Johns Hopkins, by birth-control pioneer Gregory Pincus, and by a team in Japan demonstrated that as life draws to its close, DHEA levels have gone down to about 5 percent of what they were at age 25.

Biochemist Arthur G. Schwartz of Temple University's Fels Research Institute in Philadelphia has helped show that DHEA may be effective in preventing several forms of cancer, as well as autoimmune reactions, diabetes, and obesity. This naturally produced hormone is one of our body's greatest anti-aging agents, and there is great excitement in neurobiology laboratories around the country. It is clear that we are closer than ever before to finding the chemical keys that will allow us to stay more alert and more retentive longer.

As I stated earlier, the older you are, the less DHEA you have. At the age of 80, your body produces only 10–20 percent of the DHEA it produced in the second decade of life. Studies have shown a direct relationship between blood levels of DHEA and the inhibition of many diseases.[1]

If you have high levels of DHEA you are far less likely to:

- develop atherosclerosis (and suffer from cardiovascular disease).

- develop malignant tumors (and generate cancer).

- lose insulin sensitivity (and acquire diabetes).

- suffer a decline in mental function (and lapse into dementia, Alzheimer's or Parkinson's disease, or stroke).

Because the above-mentioned disease states are the principal benchmarks of aging, DHEA may be the best biomarker of aging and longevity. Other conditions for which DHEA may be beneficial include autoimmune diseases, osteoporosis, Epstein-Barr viral infections, bacterial infections, memory loss and learning disabilities, chronic fatigue syndrome, AIDS (because of its immune impact), menopause, emotional instability, depression, stress, herpes 2 infections, and more.

Now let us take a look at the potential benefits of DHEA, category by category.

Immune System Enhancement

DHEA protects against bacterial and viral infections. Some of these are lethal viral coxsackie B enterovirus and another herpes virus type 2, enterococcus faecalis infections.

Although most major adrenocortical hormones cause immune suppression, DHEA has prevented death from infection with two different types of viruses and a fatal streptococcus infection. It is believed that

---

1   N. Orentreich, J. L. Brind, R. L. Rizer, et al, "Age changes and sex differences in serum dehydroepiandrosterone sulfate concentrations throughout adulthood," *Journal of Clinical Endocrinology* 59 (1984): 551–555.

DHEA stimulates T-cells, B-cells, and machrophages by interfering with glucocorticoid immunosuppression.[2] Scientists believe that DHEA modifies host-resistance mechanisms, but does not affect virus itself.

Regulation of Interleukin-2 Production

The immune system's T-cells contain a specific DHEA receptor. DHEA is believed to regulate the production of interleukin-2, and this may be yet another mechanism by which it improves immune function. A drug-induced suppression of T-cells, B-cells, and antibody production in rats were all reversed after administration of DHEA.[3]

DHEA and AIDS

Several studies have shown the ability of DHEA to reduce replication of the AIDS (HIV-1) virus. Clinical trials are underway for the use of DHEA as an adjunct HIV therapy. Abnormally low blood levels of DHEA are associated with increased progression of HIV infection.[4]

DHEA's Anticancer Effects

Epidemiologic studies indicate that the risk of developing a wide variety of cancers is directly related to the serum or urinary levels of DHEA or DHEA sulfate.[5] In laboratory studies, DHEA has prevented the occurrence of many different types of spontaneous and chemically induced tumors, including chemically induced adenocarcinoma of the colon, lung cancer, skin cancer, and spontaneous, viral-induced breast cancer.

Among the different types of cancers associated with low levels of DHEA are gastric cancer, prostate cancer, bladder cancer, and breast

---

2 R. M. Loria, W. Regelson, D. A. Padgett, "Immune response facilitation and resistance to virus and bacterial infections with dehydroepiandrosterone (DHEA)." In *The Biologic Role of Dehydroepiandrosterone.* Kalimi M. Regelson W., eds (New York: Walter de Gruyter 1990), 107–130.

3 K. R. Rasmussen, et al, "Effects of Dexamethasone and Dehydroepiandrosterone in Immunosuppressed Rats Infected with Cryptosporidium Parvum." *Journal of Protozoology* 38(6) (1991): 1575–1595.

4 E. Henderson, J. Y. Yang, A. Schwartz, "Dehydroepiandrosterone (DHEA) and synthetic DHEA analogs are Modest Inhibitors of HIV-I IIIB Replication." *AIDS Res. Human Retroviruses* 8(5)(1992): 625–631.

5 L. L. Pashko, et al, "Inhibition of 7, 12-dimethylbenz(a) Anthracene-induced Skin Papilomas and Carcinomas by Dehydroepiandrosterone and 3-beta-methylandrost-5-en-17-one in mice." *Cancer Res* 45(1) (1985): 164–66.

cancer. Several researchers believe that the effects of DHEA, particularly its antiproliferative effect, will ultimately be understood through its regulation of cytokines. Cytokines are bioregulatory substances, related to mammary tumor growth.

The levels of DHEA-S found in the breast fluid of some normal women exceeds plasma levels by 50 to 1,000 times. For this reason, there has been some concern that its conversion to estrogen might promote tumor growth. Animal studies have shown that DHEA can both block and stimulate mammary tumor growth. It has also been suggested that in humans a two-disease concept may apply (i.e., DHEA may act as both a promoter and suppressor of breast tumors) for pre- and postmenopausal women, derived from the ratios of DHEA/androstenedione. More studies must be done to clarify this duality.

Lower Cancer Rates in Certain Populations

The hypothesis that DHEA inhibits fat formation through reduced activity of the enzyme G6PDH is often studied as a possible mechanism for the anticancer benefits of DHEA. Adding weight to this argument is the data on hereditary carriers of G6PDH deficiency, such as Mediterrean Sephardic Jews, Greeks, and Sardinians, and a G6PD deficiency mutation common in people of African descent. One study reported lower cancer rates in Israelis of North African and Asian descent.[6]

Because of the similarity of DHEA to other sex hormones, there has been some concern that it might be implicated as a possible cause of prostate enlargement, but this has been found not to be the case.

Thymus Gland Protection

The thymus gland regulates T-cells, the immune system's principal "detectives" and "killers." Immune function normally declines with advancing age. Thymic involution, the shrinkage and incapacitation of the thymus gland, is associated with increased susceptibility to bacterial

---

6   G. B. Gordon, et al, "Serum Levels of Dehydroepiandrosterone and Dehydroepiandrosterone Sulfate and the Risk of Developing Gastric Cancer," *Cancer Epidemiological Biomarkers Prev* 2(1) (1993): 33–35.

infections, viral infections, cancers, and other types of diseases. DHEA protects thymic function by slowing shrinkage of the thymus gland.[7] In one controlled study, the immunosuppressive impact of dexamethasone, a synthetic glucocorticoid, was successfully antagonized by DHEA. Compared with controls, pretreatment with DHEA also resulted in significantly lessened dexamethasone-induced thymic atrophy.

DHEA's Anti-Atherosclerosis Effects

In hypercholesterolemic rabbits receiving heart transplants, the chronic administration of DHEA significantly retarded the progression of atherosclerosis. There was even a greater reduction in atherosclerotic rabbits who did not undergo heart transplants.[8] In rabbits whose arteries were damaged to encourage the formation of atherosclerotic plaque, DHEA reduced plaque by almost 50 percent over controls in inverse proportion to the level of serum DHEA. This finding is especially important to those who have undergone coronary bypass surgery, because grafted blood vessels are especially susceptible to new atherosclerotic formation.

Acute heart attacks are associated with low levels of DHEA and high density lipoproten (HDL). DHEA was able to prevent certain induced hypertension in rats. In a study spanning nearly two decades, men's DHEA-S levels were found to be lower in patients who died of coronary heart disease than in controls.[9]

Postmenopausal Hormone Replacement Therapy

A recent study in eight postmenopausal women concluded that DHEA may add to the benefits of estrogen therapy. The fact that DHEA protects against neoplasia, osteoporosis, and cardiac disease suggests that DHEA should be effective in treating the decline in function due

---

7 K. L. Blauer, M. Poth, W. M. Rogers, E. W. Bernton, "Dehydroepiandrosterolle Antagonizes the Suppressive Effects of Dexamethasone on Lymphocyte Proliferation," *Endocrinology*, 129(6) (1991): 3174–3179.

8 D. M. Eich, J. E. Nestler, D. E. Johnson, G. N. Dworkin, D. Ko, A. S. Wechsler, M. L. Hess, "Inhibition of Accelerated Coronary Atherosclerosis with Dehydroepiandrosterone in the Heterotopic Rabbit Model of Cardiac Transplantation," *Circulation* 87(1)(1993): 261–269.

9 A. Z. LaCroix, K. Yano, D. M. Reed, "Dehydroepiandrosterone Sulfate, Incidence of Myocardial Infarction, and Extent of Atherosclerosis in Men," *Circulation* 86(5) (1992): 1529–1535.

to menopause.[10] The use of the estrogen-receptor blocking hormone melatonin is also suggested for women undergoing estrogen replacement therapy.

Treating Dementia and Alzheimer's Disease

When circulating levels of DHEA-S were studied in 86 patients with Alzheimer's disease and multi-infarct dementia, Alzheimer's patients had lower serum levels than the controls. It was concluded that DHEA may relieve amnesia that contributes to dementia or is caused by it.[11]

Other studies have shown that DHEA and DHEA-S levels are exceedingly low at ages when the incidence of Alzheimer's disease begins to increase markedly. DHEA may play a significant role in maintaining the function of neuronal cells, and DHEA supplementation may prevent neuronal loss and/or damage, thus slowing the progress of Alzheimer's disease.

Cognition, Memory, and Learning

The exploration of DHEA's impact on memory and cognition is quite recent. Of primary note are the age-related declines in circulating brain levels of DHEA that can be correlated with declining levels of potassium channel functions.

Even small amounts of DHEA and DHEA-S were found to lessen amnesia and enhance long-term memory in mice. In vitro studies have shown that small concentrations of DHEA can enhance neuronal and glial survival in the brain cells of a mouse. Therefore, the conclusion may be that DHEA compounds might help in the treatment of neurodegenerative memory disorders in humans.[12]

---

10 J. E. Buster, et al, "Postmenopausal Steroid Replacement with Micronized Dehydroepiandrosterone: preliminary Oral Bioavailability and Dose Proportionality Studies," *American Journal of Obstetrics & Gynecology* 166(4)(1992): 1163–8.

11 B. Nasman, T. Olsson, T. Backstrom, S. Eriksson, K. Grankvist, M. Viitanen, M. Bucht, "G. Serum dehydroepiandrosterone sulfate in Alzheimer's disease and in multi-infarct dementia," *Bio Psychiatry*, 30(7) (1991): 684–690.

12 E. Roberts, L. Bologa, J. F. Flood, G. E. Smith, "Effects of Dehydroepiandrosterone and Its Sulfate on Brain tissue in Culture and on Memory in Mice," *Brain Res* 406(1–2) (1987): 357–362.

Memory enhancement was achieved by the addition of DHEA to the water supply of mice. There was a small range of dose benefit relationship. When too little DHEA was given, memory benefits dropped off steeply.

Improved memory was found in mice in one study, even when DHEA was administered after the learning experience had occurred. DHEA improved memory retention in middle-aged and old mice to the higher levels in young mice.

It appears that even very low levels of DHEA can increase the number of neurons in the brain, as well as their ability to establish contact with other neurons, and to differentiate between them.

DHEA's Anti-Diabetic Actions

Diabetics suffer a higher incidence of cardiovascular disease than people with normal carbohydrate metabolism. Recent studies suggest that one cause of the increased cardiovascular disease in diabetics may be reduced levels of DHEA caused by high levels of insulin. DHEA's multiple anti-atherogenic effects are thus thwarted when levels are abnormally low in diabetics. Since aging and obesity are both characterized by hyperinsulinemic insulin resistance, it is quite possible that the dramatically increased incidence of mature-onset diabetes and weight gain in older adults may be caused, in part, by the precipitous decline in DHEA levels accompanying advancing age.[13]

Energy "wastage" is thought to be one of the ways that DHEA reduces body weight. In a study with rats, DHEA seemed to exert part of its antiobesity and antidiabetic effects through increased hepatic glucose oxidation and reduced gluconeogenesis.

Obesity and diabetes are characterized by high levels of gluconeogenesis, occurring in spite of increased levels of insulin. In both insulin-resistant mutant mice and in normal aging mice, DHEA increases sensitivity to insulin, thereby increasing the effects of this important hormone.

---

13 J. E. Nestler, J. N. Clore, W. G. Blackard, "Dehydro-epiandrosterone: the 'Missing Link' Between Hyperinsulinemia and Atherosclerosis?" *FASEB Journal* 6(12) 1992): 3073–3075.

DHEA also ameliorates the effects of diabetes in disease-prone mice. Rats genetically predisposed to diabetes do not develop the disease when given DHEA, nor do they suffer damage to "islet cells" which produce insulin in the pancreas when given DHEA. Some clinicians have reported that DHEA treatment reduces the need for insulin in humans.

DHEA's Antiobesity Effects

One of the most striking effects of DHEA is its ability to induce weight loss in laboratory animals, even when these animals are given as much food as they want. This remarkable finding by Dr. Arthur Schwartz of Temple University Medical School in the 1980s produced tremendous interest in the possibility of using DHEA as a weight-loss therapy in humans. Recent research has begun to show how DHEA exerts its extraordinary weight-loss effects.

A recent study in diabetes-prone rats indicates that one of DHEA's weight-reducing mechanisms may operate through the increase of serotonin levels in the hypothalamus region of the brain, thereby increasing the release of cholecytokinin (CCK), the satiation hormone. CCK reduces one's desire for foods by creating a feeling of fullness. DHEA-fed rats showed an increase in serotonin levels in the hypothalamus, which was associated with increased CCK activity, reduced food intake and lower body fat.

DHEA also is believed to produce its antiobesity effects by antiglucocorticoid activity.[14] In this study, DHEA blocked the activity of the glucocorticoid-induced enzymes, tyrosine aminotransferase, and ornithine decarboxylase in genetically obese rats, leading to substantial weight loss in these animals.

Among the other mechanisms proposed to explain DHEA's ability to induce weight loss and fat reduction are its effects on lipogenesis, substrate cycling, peroxisome proliferation, mitochondrial respiration, protein synthesis, and thyroid hormone function. Beyond its inhibition of

---

14   B. E. Wright, J. R. Portei, E. S. Browne, "Antiglucocorticoid Action of Dehydroepiandrosterone in Young Obese Zucker Rats." *International Journal of Obesity* 16(8) (1992): 579–583.

fat synthesis and deposition, DHEA operates via mechanisms which help to *expend* energy rather than store it for future use.

DHEA can prevent obesity in genetically predisposed mice. When given DHEA, the body weights of genetically obese mice dropped to that of lean mice independent of any alteration in food intake. Even middle-aged, genetically obese mice were thin after being given DHEA. Rats, whose obesity had been induced by a high-calorie diet, lost weight rapidly when treated with DHEA. DHEA also produced lipid and insulin-lowering effects.

Antiobesity Effects in Humans

DHEA was given to five male, normal-weight subjects at a dose of 1600 mg per day, divided into four doses. After 28 days, with diet and physical activity remaining normal, four of the five exhibited a mean body fat decrease of 31 percent with no overall weight change. This meant that their fat loss was balanced by a gain in muscle mass characteristic of youth! At the same time, their LDL levels fell by 7.5 percent to confer protection against cardiovascular disease.[15]

Effect Upon Depression

Subjects suffering from unipolar depression were given various forms of pharmacotherapy and behavioral therapy. The DHEA-S levels of 47 subjects showed a positive correlation with rating scale improvement as their depression was relieved.[16]

Life Extension

Aging in humans is characterized by reduced control over the production of cytokine inerleukin-6 (IL-6), thought to play an important role in controlling abnormal cell proliferation. The loss of control over IL-6

15 J. E. Nestler, C. O. Barlascini, J. N. Clore, W. G. Blackard, "Dehydroepiandosterone Reduces Serum Low Density Lipoprotein Levels and Body Fat but Does Not Alter Insulin Sensitivity in Normal Men." *Journal of Clinical Endocrinology & Metabolism* 66(1) (1988): 57–61.

16 G. D. Tollefson, E. Haus, M. J. Garvey, M. Evans, W. B. Tuason, "24 Hour Urinary Dehydroepiandrosterone Sulfate in Unipolar Depression Treated with Cognitive and/or Pharmacotherapy." *Annals of .Clinical Psychiatry* 2(1) (1990): 39–46.

has been shown to be preventable or even reversible with DHEA-S treatment in old mice. When treated, these mice also exhibited lower than normal levels of serum amyloid-P substance, serum Ig, and tissue specific autoantibodies, compared with untreated, aged controls. Because each of these measures is aging related, these findings provide evidence that DHEA may help to slow "normal" aging.[17]

The antibody response of mice to a vaccine was found to decline with age at Kentucky University's Sanders-Brown Center on Aging. Yet, DHEA significantly enhanced their splenic immune responses and the discrepancy was reversed.

Studies have shown that DHEA can increase lifespans by 50 percent in laboratory animals. DHEA levels were found to be inversely related to death due to all causes in men over 50. Mice did not age as rapidly when fed DHEA, and maintained their youthful hair color and sleekness, compared with the graying, coarsening hair of the control animals.[18]

DHEA is found in great concentrations throughout the brain and body. It is synthesized from cholesterol primarily in the adrenal cortex system. DHEA is sulfated readily to DHEA-S that is mostly interchangeable with and reconvertible to DHEA. A generation ago, DHEA and its sulfate (DHEA-S) were seen only as links in the production of sex hormones, but that has changed dramatically, as a growing body of evidence has emerged about how this prodigious hormone functions in the body.

DHEA follows two metabolic pathways: the first is via the liver circulation, and the second involves DHEA's conversion in the skin tissue where it is believed to exert a stimulating effect on the immune system. The nice thing about its discovery is that it biochemically supports the consciousness and PNI studies that illustrate our ability to slow down the aging process, look younger, and live longer and better, naturally.

---

17 R. A. Daynes, et al, "Altered Regulation of IL-6 Production with Normal Aging: Possible Linkage to the Age-associated Decline in Dehydroepiandrosterone and its Sulfated Derivative." *Journal of Immunology* 150(12)(1993): 5219–5230.

18 W. Regelson, R. Loria, M. Kalimi, "Hormonal Intervention: "Buffer Hormones" or "State Dependency," The Role of Dehydroepiandrosterone (DHEA), Thyroid Hormone, Estrogen and Hypohysectomy in Aging." *Annals of New York Academy of Science* 521 (1988): 260–273.

THEORIES ON AGING

There is no shortage of theories on aging. The National Institute on Aging lists fourteen different theories, ranging from wear-and-tear, rate-of-living, and error catastrophe, to metabolic, endocrine, free-radical, somatic mutation, collagen, programmed senescene, cross-linking, immunological, redundant message, codon restriction, or transcriptional event theories.

George Burns starred in *The Sunshine Boys* at 79, and was still performing at 99.

Many scientists look to DNA (the genetic code of all of our cells) as the cause of aging. Because of exposure to toxins, chemicals, and ultraviolet light filtering through the skin, these complex chains of information-carrying chemicals may break, twist, become transposed, or otherwise get out of order. When they do, the cells are not able to pass along their genetic blueprints accurately, and key chemical reactions within the body's cells begin to break down. When enough of these cells break down, the changes accumulate into serious deficits that weaken whole organs.

Faulty enzymes constitute another aging theory. These defective enzymes, instead of maintaining the well-ordered cellular chemical production lines that Nature designed, make our cells start to look like a crazed, disorderly factory floor, turning out too much of some things and not enough of others.

The "error catastrophe theory" suggests that defective proteins in the body's cells accumulate into an intracellular chemical soup that interferes with the cells' proper biochemical tasks and thus weakens them. If we could control the DNA, all the DNA, then we should be able to keep those assembly lines moving...maybe not forever, but for an impressively long time.

The most compelling of the many aging theories advanced by cell biologists is called the "free-radical" theory. Free radicals are very reactive chemical by-products that are created as oxygen is burned as fuel in our cells. Chemically, they are molecules out of electrical balance. The only way they know to rebalance themselves is to steal an electron belonging to another molecule, thereby unbalancing it, and so the chain reaction goes on, unleashing all sorts of havoc.

As they react explosively with many of your cells' natural chemicals, these free-radical reactions can inflict severe damage on the fragile equilibrium of the cells. Free radicals destroy key cell enzymes, fats, and proteins. They can interfere with the delicate mechanism of DNA and RNA that is responsible for cell division. They can trigger inflammation, damage lung cells and blood vessels, and lead to mutations, cell destruction, degenerative diseases, and even cancer. When enough of that happens, there is a cascade of biological damage. The cumulative levels of oxidation radicals put millions, even billions, of cells out of commission. Their numbers increase as we age.

One school of thought, based on the breakthrough research of the eminent biologist Dr. Denham Harman of the University of Nebraska's College of Medicine, believes that the cumulative effect of free-radical damage is the root of cell aging. "Chances are 99 percent that free radicals are the basis for aging," says biochemist Harman, the father of free-radical theory. "Aging is the ever-increasing accumulation of changes caused or contributed to by free radicals."[1]

---

1   Denham Harman, Free radical theory on Aging: Dietary Implications," *American Journal of Clinical Nutrition* (August, 1972).

Dr. Harman found that vitamin E effectively neutralizes these "free radicals." By feeding vitamin E to aged rats, Harman found not only that the "old-timers" were mentally and physically rejuvenated but that their life spans were increased by a full 30 percent. In a similar experiment performed by Richard Hochschild of the University of California, the life spans of treated rats were extended by an incredible 49 percent! In human terms this means a potential extension of life span to 180 years. Hochschild also found that his rats were rejuvenated and retained their good health until the very hour of their deaths.[2]

These scientists blame free radicals for many common degenerative diseases: arthritis, diabetes, hardening of the arteries, heart and kidney ailments, Parkinson's disease, even cataracts. Although scientists may disagree whether the aging culprit is DNA, free radicals, defective cell enzymes, or some combination of these and other factors, what links all of them is a belief that losing our youthful vigor is a process of entropy, the result of the wear of existence. They tell us it is when our cells grow increasingly snarled, jumbled, and generally muddled with chemical clutter that we start to look, act, and feel old.

The second major school of theorists says there is more to aging than mere entropy. The human body is programmed to self-destruct, and the code to do so is written in our genes. Studies by Dr. W. Donner Denckla at Harvard University have shown that the human pituitary gland secretes a "death hormone" which interferes with the body's ability to utilize thyroxine. Thyroxine is a hormone produced by the thyroid which directly controls the rate of cellular metabolism.[3]

This hormone is DECO—the aging or death, or antithyroid hormone, or family of hormones, presumed to be the regulator of the genetic clock of aging—that Denckla was trying so hard to isolate, purify, and synthesize over the years. Russia's V. V. Frolkis corroborated Denckla's

---

2   Richard Hochschild, "Effect of Dimethylaminoethanol on the Life Span of Senile Male A/J Rats." (*Experimental Gerontology*, vol. 8, 1973).

3   W. D. Denckla, "Searching for the 'Death' Hormone," interview in *Anti-Aging News* (October, 1981).

work by reporting that as we age the blood contains increasing concentrations of substances that inhibit the functioning of the pancreatic hormones, much as Denckla believes that DECO inhibits the functioning of the thyroid hormone. Frolkis also, quite independently, notes the decline with age of the body's ability to bind thyroxine.[4]

A number of critical imbalances could very well be explained by a decrease in cellular thyroxine. Such destructive changes as the generation of more free radicals lead to more cross-linkages, more somatic mutations, more error catastrophes. More toxins may be produced, leaving more cellular garbage than the cell can dispose of, and this would lead to some of the changes we associate with aging.

Autoimmune response could also result from this decrease in efficiency of the immune cells themselves, worsening the general disruption. DECO may act on the thymic cells to cut down production of thymosin and other thymic hormones (perhaps even causing the shrinkage of the thymus, which occurs in everyone at a relatively early age), further impairing immunologic function and increasing the risk of cancer and lethal infection. The aging or death hormones might even operate principally at the level of genetic on/off switching.

NIA's Richard Veech, William Regelson of the Medical College of Virginia at Richmond, Richard Cutler of NIA's GRC/Baltimore, Robert Bolla of the University of Missouri in St. Louis, several Soviet scientists, and Australian Arthur Everitt, who, along with Denckla, has pioneered this research frontier, all share Denckla's belief in a brain-based hormonal clock of aging. USC's Caleb Finch is convinced that one or more hormones must play a large part in aging, and that certain small areas of the primitive brain must be an important part of the clockwork.

The possibility of genetic programming may explain why the human species seems to have a fixed upper age of about 120 years. That presumably represents the maximum age our genes are "set" to. At one

---

4   V. V. Frolkis, "Regulation and Adaptation Processes in Aging," *The Main Problems of Soviet Gerontology* (Kiev, 1972).

time it was believed that human cells could divide indefinitely. Now it is known that adult cells divide only about 50 times and then mysteriously die. Gerontologist Leonard Hayflick, Ph.D., thinks there are trillions of such clocks inside each of us. Based on painstaking and ingenious experiments with cell cultures, he proposes that we have such a clock in the nucleus of each of the body's cells. At a certain point the clock stops running, and that point, chemically set before birth, varies for different species, Hayflick theorizes.[5] However, this theory does not explain why identical twins do not die within a year of each other.

UCLA's preeminent research pathologist Roy Walford believes that immune system decline is probably controlled by a group of genes called the major histocompatibility complex (MHC). The MHC may affect breakage and repair of DNA, the levels of free radicals, even the pace at which our tissues develop and regenerate.

It is quite possible that none of the theories of aging is really wrong. The designated events do undoubtedly occur, and they are usually responsible, to some degree, for other kinds of damage. If it were to go on long enough, any event or process could eventually kill us. The free-radical theory may unify all the wear-and-tear theories by encompassing them in a manner that can explain the claims of each.

Techniques such as two-dimensional electrophoresis and high-pressure liquid chromatography make indexes of our proteins. Many scientists are confident that one day we will have mapped all our genes and indexed all our proteins—found ways, in fact, to do it on an individual basis, since no two of us are identical. The health professional of the future may simply retrieve this information from their computer, along with our unique biochemical pathways and other individualized information, so that they may utilize this knowledge, not merely to treat diseases, but to maintain us in an optimal state of health for a much longer time.

If you can increase your life expectancy from the seventy-five years that the statisticians tell us is now the norm even halfway up to the

5 Leonard Haylflick, "Recent Advances in the Cell Biology of Aging," *Mechanisms of Aging and Development*, Vol. 1, 1980).

theoretical current maximum of 120 years (97.5), you would lengthen your life by 30 percent. Linus Pauling, three-time Nobel Prize-winning biochemist, estimates in *How to Live Longer and Feel Better* that using health measures presently available, we can increase our life expectancy from 25 to 35 years.[6]

Since the beginning of the twentieth century, people in developed countries have already added an astounding 28 years to their average life span. I see no logical reason for this extension of our life not to expand even further.

We must remember that such an increase in longevity requires no fundamental change in scientific understanding and no major conceptual breakthroughs. It is interesting to note that it doesn't necessarily matter which of the many theories ultimately prove right.

By following the recommendations in part II, you will eliminate risk factors and unnecessary toxins from your life; you will give your cells a chance to rebuild themselves. Your goal is to eliminate the factors that could prematurely cut short your life long before its true biological deadline. By doing so, you will let your body take advantage of the wonderful longevity that Nature originally designed for it.

---

6   Linus Pauling, *How to Live Longer and Feel Better* (New York: Avon, 1987).

CONSCIOUSNESS
AND AGING

Albert Einstein once wrote: "Everyone who is seriously involved in the pursuit of science becomes convinced that a Spirit is manifest in the Laws of the Universe—a Spirit vastly superior to that of man, and one in the face of which we, with our modest powers, must feel humble."[1]

French designer Coco Chanel retired at 55, then went back to work at 71.

We often hear people say, "how *old* are you? Or "you are only as *old* as you think you are." I prefer to say, "You are as *young* as you think you are." My point here is not just semantics. Your mind is the most powerful weapon in your arsenal against premature aging.

The relatively new science of psychoneuroimmunology (PNI) measures the connection between our mind (attitudes, beliefs, and emotions) and the health and vitality of our organs. Unraveling the mind-body connection is the goal of PNI.

PNI findings have demonstrated:

- Grieving, stress, and depression have all been proven to lower our body's immunological fighter cells dramatically.

---

1   Helen Dukas and Banesh Hoffmann, eds. *Albert Einstein, The Human Side* (Princeton: Princeton University Press, 1979), p. 33.

- Brain chemicals that regulate happiness, sex drive, mental functioning, sleep, depression, aggression, and all of our other brain functions have been found to activate specific immune fighters such as scavenger cells, T killer cells, antibody-producing cells, and immune boosters like interferon and interleukin-2.

- Our immune system's strength reflects our emotional and mental coping mechanisms. Lifestyle and psychological stresses can weaken our immune defenses, increase the likelihood of catching infections, and raise our risk for many kinds of diseases.

- Animals given control over their environment fight off tumors better and live longer than animals with no control.

- Institutionalized people who have more control over their lives show dramatic improvements in overall health, even reversing bodily changes due to aging.

- George Washington University physicians found that patients can use mental imagery to change the levels of certain immune cells necessary to fight cancer.

- By programming themselves with mental-relaxation tools, people can lower blood pressure and reduce the frequency of heart-rhythm abnormalities.

- Research at Vanderbilt University Medical Center shows that patients who are programmed to expect a slow recovery after surgery exhibit more physical problems than those who expect to leave the hospital quickly.

Consciousness is the true foundation of all we know and perceive. Etymologically, the word "consciousness" derives from the Latin *scire* (to know) and *cum* (with). Consciousness is "to know with." To me, this term implies nonlocal knowing; we cannot know somebody (or our body) without sharing a nonlocal connection with that person or our biological structure.

The beliefs that you hold, whether deliberately chosen or indoctrinated, create a model for interpreting and structuring reality. This model is sometimes called a *personal reality paradigm*. I call it your viewpoint.

If you want to take a very broad look at consciousness, you will discover that it consists of viewpoint and some attendant ability to reason—meaning to observe, integrate, predict, and act. Viewpoint determines how you see the world and how you see yourself. Not liking something is a viewpoint. Even when you feel your opinion is on rock-solid ground, there is still a little suspicion that maybe someone else might feel differently. (Of course, you are right, and they are wrong.)

Protecting a viewpoint is a refusal to see something in a certain way. Have you ever heard someone say, "Everyone's entitled to their own viewpoint," or "I'm not going to change my viewpoint just because you disagree"? Yes, these are viewpoints too—fixed viewpoints.

When people lock themselves into certain viewpoints, they lock themselves out of other viewpoints. As they limit how they are willing to look at something, they also limit their ability to observe, integrate, predict, and act. Their ability to relate to others is limited. Their ability to handle life is limited. Their ability to cope with change is limited.

Sometimes a little thing, like showing someone how to deliberately change his or her viewpoint without being struck dumb on the spot, can produce a remarkable recovery of their zest for life. Problems disappear and opportunities reappear. It's a simple act that has magical consequences. One of these opportunities is the slowing down of the aging process.

The easiest way to change something is to change your viewpoint. This does not always result in a change in the world, but it will place you in the optimum position should you wish to make a change in the world. From the eternal stillness of source, one creates each successive moment of existence, as it was, as it is, and as it will be. All joys, all sorrows, all opportunities, and all limitations roll forth into creation from this stillness here and now. Understanding that you are the convergent point of every reality is true perspective.

We all share an overwhelming intuition that our mind is separate from our body. There is also the conflicting intuition that mind and body are the same—as when we are in bodily pain. Additionally, we intuit that we have a self separate from the world, an individual self that is conscious of what is going on in our minds and bodies, a self that wills (freely?) some of the actions of the body. The philosophers of the mind-body problem examine these intuitions.

First, there are philosophers who propose that our intuition of a mind (and consciousness) separate from the body is right. These are the dualists. Others deny dualism; they are the monists. There are two schools of monists. One school, the material monists, feels that body is primary and that mind and consciousness are but epiphenomena of the body. The second school, the monistic idealists, declare that consciousness is prior to experience. It is without an object and without a subject.

This state of being we call consciousness, according to the monistic idealists, is prior and unconditioned. It is all there is. The mind and body are merely an epiphenomena of consciousness; it is the true foundation of all we know and perceive. Consciousness, through our self-reference, creates material reality. The new physics (Quantum physics) mathematically and experimentally supports the monistic idealists. In Western culture, particularly in recent times, the material monists have dominated the monist school. In the East, on the other hand, monistic idealism has remained a force.

After spending more than ten years corroborating the mind-body effects of transcendental meditation (TM), in 1978 Robert Keith Wallace decided to study aging. His hypothesis focused on the premise that if the meditators could counter the effects of stress and pressure through this simple mind-body relaxation discipline, they could slow down the aging process.[2]

We define biological age as how well a person functions in comparison to the norms of the whole population. This biological age is a far

2   R. K. Wallace, et al, "Effects of the TM and TM-Sidhi Program on the Aging Process," *International Journal of Neuroscience*, 16 (1982): 53–58.

more accurate measure of the aging process than chronological age. The three variables Wallace tested were near-point vision (the ability to see objects close up), blood pressure, and acute hearing. Since all three steadily deteriorate as the body ages biologically, the variables served well as markers of aging.

There is no established scientific evidence that aging is a normal process. Not surprisingly, Wallace observed that the meditators were biologically younger than their chronological age. It must be pointed out here that since hypnosis and meditation are both alpha brain-wave states (and are identical neurologically), the conclusions drawn from these TM studies also apply to the use of hypnosis.

Wallace's results showed that a female subject was 20 years younger biologically than her chronological age. The amount of time a group meditated had dramatic effects on their biological age. Those who meditated five years or more averaged 12 years younger biologically. The group that practiced meditation less than five years averaged five years younger.

An English study reported that each year of meditation took off one year of aging. Wallace was impressed by the fact that older subjects had results equal to the younger ones. A typical 60-year-old meditating five years or more would have the physiology of a 48-year-old.

It is interesting to note that the subjects in Wallace's study were *not* trying to age more slowly. By using consciousness principles, these subjects removed the only barrier to the aging process. A 1986 Blue Cross-Blue Shield insurance study based on two thousand meditators in Iowa showed that they were much healthier than the American population as a whole in seventeen major areas of serious disease, both mental and physical.

In the Blue Cross-Blue Shield study, meditators were hospitalized 50 percent less often for all kinds of tumors and 87 percent less often than nonmeditators for heart disease. Reductions in clinical depression or for disorders of the digestive tract or respiratory system were also observed. This lower morbidity exhibited by TM practitioners is most significant.

No longer must we assume that healthy people will deteriorate as they grow older. Many senile symptoms once thought permanent are now shown to be reversible. The previously noted signs of "aging" may be merely the by-product of isolation, dehydration, poor nutrition, and other factors.

Choice is now recognized as an element of aging. Wallace showed that people do not age by bits and pieces, but as whole human beings. Expanding our consciousness by such techniques as hypnosis and meditation opens up our awareness to the point where anything is possible. We now have direct evidence that consciousness controls aging.

Programming a slowing down of the aging process is one development stemming from this awareness expansion. Using the alpha technique stops distracting mental activity, and cellular activity is altered. Most of us have been acculturated to expect deterioration with advancing years, and that is exactly what we get. By changing this programming we can now get to the heart of the aging process—the DNA. We will discuss this in greater detail in chapter 13.

Charles Alexander of Harvard visited three retirement homes outside Boston and trained groups of residents in mind-body alpha techniques. The meditators, all 80 years old or more, scored highest on mental health, learning ability, and low blood pressure, all of which usually decline with age. The residents stated they felt better and younger. Three years later Alexander returned to one retirement home and was informed that 24 percent of the control group who had not learned meditation had died. All of the meditators, however, were still living.[3]

The term "consciousness" was introduced to American psychology by William James. He contended that beyond the range of normal waking consciousness lies the possibility of special or exceptional states that are completely "discontinuous" with discursive thought.[4] Maharishi

---

3   C. N. Alexander, et al, "Transcendal Meditation, Mindfulness and Longevity: An Experimental Study with the Elderly," *Journal of Personal Social Psychology,* 57 (1989): 950–964.

4   W. James, *The Principles of Psychology* (New York: Henry Holt, 1890).

Mahesh Yogi, who introduced TM as a simple mental technique derived from the Vedic tradition of India, proposed that through this procedure, a "fourth major state of consciousness" can be regularly experienced.

This fourth state is referred to in Maharishi's Vedic psychology as transcendental consciousness because it is said to transcend or be discontinuous with the three ordinary states of waking, dreaming, and sleep. This state is also traditionally described as "pure" consciousness and it is the state I use when I guide the patient to the superconscious mind level during a superconscious mind tap (see chapter 13).

Consciousness and the New Physics

In order for there to be consciousness, there must be choice. The new physics clearly demonstrates that we choose between alternatives and this helps create and shape our reality. Since there must be mind to make these choices, there must be consciousness.

Quantum physicists mathematically demonstrate that an event must be observed to be a component of reality. Our entire universe is a product of our mind. One only needs to change one's mind to alter this reality. The world appears as a by-product of this form of mental gymnastics. The new physics tells us that it is our observations that actually determine and shape events in our life. We are not mere observers, nor can we separate ourselves from the events we see.

J. S. Hagelin has demonstrated that there are close structural parallels between the technical properties of the unified field of quantum field theory and the descriptions by both ancient and modern meditators of the field of pure consciousness experienced when conscious awareness settles into its "least excited state," the unified field of pure consciousness, which can be directly experienced by the human nervous system to achieve higher levels of health and well-being.[5]

---

5 J. S. Hagelin, "Is consciousness the Unified Field? A Field Theorist's Perspective." *Modern Science and Vedic Science,* 1(1), (1987): 28–87.

Conscious mental activity can affect the things of the physical world—including the organs, tissues, and cells that compose our bodies. Mind is an irrefutably genuine factor in the process by which health and disease unfold themselves, and this includes the process of aging.

Nobel Prize laureate physicist Eugene Wigner stated that if mind could *not* affect the physical world, but was only affected by it, this would be the only known example in modern physics of such a one-way interaction. In modern physics, one-way interactions are not known to occur.

The "will to live" is a good example of consciousness principles. Some patients exhibit an aggressive, tenacious, and argumentative demeanor. They follow instructions poorly, do not get along with doctors and nurses, and seem to defy their illnesses. This is a sharp contrast to the passive, meek, compliant person who is typically referred to as a good patient. The patient with the will to live frequently outlives his or her prognosis. Is this patient giving us evidence that consciousness affects the physical world?

Another unpredictable principle in medicine is "the natural course of a disease." Some patients die within a few weeks of being diagnosed with cancer, while others live for years with a malignancy. Spontaneous cures have been reported with cancer. This is simply not supposed to happen. Is consciousness at work again?

The placebo effect is another illustration of consciousness. Patients who think they are taking some specific medication or miracle drug are cured when, in reality, all they took was a sugar pill. Biofeedback experiments illustrate that variability in many human physiological responses is known to be highly susceptible to the impact of consciousness.

We must look beyond the euphemisms of "human variability," "the placebo response," and "the natural course of the disease," and attempt to dissect the effect of human consciousness on specific disease and aging processes.

---

5   E. Wigner, *Physical Science and Human Values* (Princeton: Princeton University Press, 1947).

Several mathematical models in quantum physics explain the influence of a patient's consciousness on the physical world (the body). Our body only ages beyond our control if you accept the programming of conventional society and medicine. This collective conditioning must be broken in order to slow down and reverse the aging process.

Resolving the consciousness problem to assist you in your new programming, consider these examples of society's paradigm, a paradigm that is absolutely incorrect:

- Mind and body are separate and independent from each other.

- Suffering is a necessary part of our world. We are mere victims of aging, sickness, and death.

- No one can escape the effects of time.

- The world is objective and completely independent of the observer. Our physical bodies are one component of this objective world.

- The world that we perceive through our five senses is a perfectly accurate depiction of our universe.

- As beings we are isolated from consciousness of others and the energy of the universe.

- Our true being is merely the sum of our body, personality, and emotions.

- Our physical body consists of physical matter isolated from each other and from other forces in our universe.

- The material world is the determiner of our reality. Consciousness is explained as a physiological process.

- Biochemistry and Neurophysiology are responsible for the entire range of human awareness.

If we accept these assumptions, time is seen as our jailor and we are its prisoners. Materialistic concepts of cynicism and defeatism completely ignore consciousness. All of our thoughts have an effect on aging. Each cognition exerts an impact on our cells. Accomplishing a desired goal can invigorate our immune system, while depression significantly compromises it.

Cancer and heart attacks can be brought on by hopelessness and despair. An act of kindness and experiences of joy extend our longevity by slowing down the process of aging. Negative memories of life stresses can be as damaging to our body and our psyche as the stress itself.

The main point I want to make here is that the process of aging is changeable. We can stop it, speed up its progress, or slow it down. Reversing Father Time is not out of the question, as some of the studies already presented demonstrated. Several hundred research findings have shown that consciousness plays a significant role in aging.

In order to make these techniques and principles more effective, a global change in view and paradigm is required, substituting new principles for the ten false assumptions described earlier (p. 65).

The new corrected principles are:

- Mind and body are intermingled. Consciousness coordinates this unity and the body acts as a receptacle for this stream of consciousness.

- We create suffering and can uncreate it. Consciousness frees us from aging, sickness, and even death.

- Time is eternal and relative. There is a space-time continuum, but linear time only exists if we accept that concept.

- Our physical world is a mere creation of our consciousness. Without an observer there is no world.

- Perception is learned and affected by our experience. We can change our world and the process of aging by altering our perception of them.

- We are the aggregate of energy impulses. All of us are connected to the energy of the universe.

- Energy and consciousness is what our bodies consist of, in essence. The physical body is a creation of our consciousness.

- Our awareness through consciousness creates the biochemistry and anatomy of our body. It is the forgetting of our true consciousness nature that results in aging.

- Consciousness is always the primary aspect of our being. Materialism is simply the creation of consciousness.

- Human awareness is a product of consciousness, not neurology or biochemistry. It is our consciousness that creates the biochemistry and other aspects of our body, including aging.

Your process of aging began to change when you read the above principles. To make this change permanent, however, you will need to incorporate this reality into your awareness and consciousness. Quantum physics has given us a solid cientific foundation for these concepts.

The techniques presented in part II will assist you on all levels to change your reality. The new physics teaches us that without an observer there is no reality. All of us create a different universe. Do not be misled by your five senses. You created them also.

Do you consider the Earth to be flat? Trusting your immediate environment would support that concept. Up until 500 yeas ago that was the accepted "fact," and statements to the contrary would have sometimes resulted in a painful death.

What we all need is a perceptual shift to slow down the aging process. You and I may live in an objective world of materialism, but if you see yourself in the world and I see a better world in myself, I may be chronologically 20 years older than you and still outlive you by several decades. This freedom from the bondage and toil of aging can only be attained by a perception shift.

Awareness can be used for positive health or to create sickness. It is a matter of programming and motivation. Your beliefs, attitudes, reactions, and assumptions will determine which path you will take.

Destructive and negative thoughts result in illness and destructive behavior. Positive and constructive cognitions have the opposite effect. It is not just your thoughts—it's also attitude, motivation, assumptions, actions, and emotions that reflect your consciousness. Do not be concerned about trying to do psychic surgery on yourself. Focus on consciousness and you are confronting the only factor that matters.

The *Tao Te Ching* states, "Whatever is flexible and flowing will tend to grow, whatever is rigid and blocked will wither and die." Change your thoughts, open up your mind, eliminate all previous prejudices, cynicism, and so on. Expect the best and become a realistic idealist. Break with fixed and negative patterns of the past that locked your mind into repeated and self-destructive patterns.

As we develop from childhood, we receive various forms of data, mostly in verbal form. Psychologists estimate that our parents alone are responsible for more than 25,000 hours of programming. This does not include conditioning we receive from teachers, peers, relatives, and television.

What you do get is "stuff" handed down from society and filtered through your family and friends. Neurosis begets neurosis. When your mother observed early signs of aging (wrinkles, a gray hair, etc.), did she panic and instill anxiety over this event? Probably so, resulting in your programming to expect and fear aging.

Let us not forget your father and grandparents. Did your father accept retirement easily? How did your grandparents react to their more obvious signs of aging? Did the latter feel useless and abandoned? Remember the discussion in chapter 4 of the supernormals in the Caucasus Mountains?

Choice always becomes restricted as a result of conditioning. A recovering alcoholic has a far different outlook when someone unaware of his or her past offers them a drink. Most people will accept or reject an alcoholic beverage depending on the time of day, occasion, or simply a whim, but for a recovering alcoholic, this is a major life choice.

Space here doesn't permit a lengthy discussion about compulsive personalities. Suffice it to say that it is the person's consciousness that was programmed to live the life of a recovering alcoholic, although some will cite a genetic argument about a predisposition to alcoholism.

A quick review of the ten correct consciousness principles will illustrate the fact that our mind (consciousness) creates the biochemistry, not the other way around. Regardless of the pleas of the recovering alcoholic, anorexic, bulimic, compulsive gambler, and perpetual procrastinator, it all boils down to the same bottom line: they live in an illusion that dictates hopelessness and helplessness.

I refer to this as the Wayne's World syndrome: "we're not worthy" (to meet Alice Cooper in Wayne's case). If you extrapolate this concept to, "I can't slow down aging," or "it's only a matter of time before I acquire heart disease or cancer" (the two most common causes of death in America), you have lost the consciousness game.

Any illusion can be broken. A mirage of an oasis seen by someone in the desert dissolves when the individual reaches the supposed location only to find that it was merely sand. Society fills us with many illusions; if we allow them to exist, we control the acceptance stage.

You can easily recognize the operation of an illusion when you sense or observe a choice that appears to be cut off. For example, you see a relative or friend grow old and die. Now death becomes real and you question your own mortality. You wonder when your time will be up and your own aging process is hastened.

Does your car break down and fall apart merely because it sees other cars wind up in the junk yard? Some say inanimate objects do possess consciousness, but that is a different book. Assume for the purpose of this discussion that the car has no consciousness. It can only respond to wear and tear, and maintenance. By not being aware of aging, it doesn't age unless we overuse it and neglect its care.

We have consciousness, and therein lies both the problem and the solution. The study of primitive societies reveals much about the way consciousness works. *The Paleolithic Prescription,* co-authored by S. Boyd Eaton, cites over 25 traditional societies throughout the world almost devoid of cancer and heart disease.[6] Due to their very different styles of conditioning, the two most associated diseases of aging have been all but eliminated. What are they doing right? Better yet, what are we Westerners doing wrong?

These anthropological investigations show that abnormal conditioning and limited choices result in "normal" aging. Eaton points out that in certain African desert societies, and in Tasmania, the Solomon Islands, and Venezuela, low blood pressure throughout life is the norm. The opposite occurs in Western Europe and the United States. Blood pressure typically rises by a few millimeters of mercury every decade and nearly half of the aged population receives treatment for high blood pressure.

The Maabans of Sudan and certain Bushman tribes in Botswana maintain excellent hearing as they age. That is not the case in America, where nearly ten percent of the population suffers from enough hearing loss to be considered disabled. A study among Tennessee college freshmen revealed that hearing loss was evidenced by 60 percent of the students.

A rise in cholesterol levels is considered a biomarker of aging in the West. Yet the Tarahumara Indians of Northern Mexico and the Tanzanian Hadzas rarely exhibit cholesterol levels of over 150. The American average is 210. These primitive societies are well protected against premature heart attacks by such low readings that remain at this level throughout their lives. The American rate naturally rises as we age because that is the way we are conditioned.

Breast cancer is very rare in Japan and China. In America one woman in nine will develop this cancer. These Asian countries also exhibit far lower colon cancer rates than those found among American men.

---

6   S. Boyd Eaton, et al., *The Paleolithic Prescription: A Program of Diet & Exercise & a Design for Living* (New York: Harper-Row, 1989).

Rates of high blood pressure, colon cancer, and heart attacks rise when Africans, Taiwanese, or Japanese populations migrate from their homeland to America. By the second generation these families exhibit the same pattern of aging as exhibited by Americans.

On the surface it would appear that the diet and lifestyle changes afforded with the move to America would explain this rise in aging diseases, but not according to David Sobel and Robert Ornstein as reported in their book, *The Healing Brain.* The Japanese males who retained strong bonds to their culture, despite their geographic move to America, continued to have low rates of heart disease.[7]

The interesting aspect of this study is that these Japanese males adopted an American diet and the cholesterol levels in their blood rose. These men attended school with fellow Japanese students, observed social ties and traditional customs and continued speaking their native language. These consciousness factors more than balanced their higher cholesterol levels and resulted in surprisingly greater resistance to cardiovascular disease. Of course, this is only surprising if you are looking for strictly medical reasons for this change, and ignore consciousness considerations.

When studies were conducted with laid-off auto workers in Michigan, consciousness factors were again demonstrated in relation to the frequency of psychosomatic symptoms. Those workers who experienced the strongest support from family, friends, and relatives during their hard times developed far less mental and physical symptoms. The opposite also held true.

Another study with pregnant women paralleled these results. Ninety-one percent of serious complications during their pregnancies were experienced by those women who felt they had little social support. This extension of consciousness simply cannot be ignored as it relates to physiological effects on our body, not the least of which its effect on the process of aging.

---

7   Robert Ornstein and David Sobel, *The Healing Brain: Breakthrough Medical Discoveries about How the Brain Keeps Us Healthy* (New York: Simon & Schuster, 1987).

We can learn quite a bit from studies such as these. If we accept society's dictum that aging is inevitable and will be characterized by heart problems, cancer, arthritis, and so on, then this victimization will continue. However, if we empower ourselves and realize that much of the aging characteristics we see are simply the result of social conditioning, then we can program out this stereotype and replace these paradigms with new beliefs of increased longevity and a qualitative lifestyle.

Our Beliefs about Aging

A belief is a philosophy that you hold to be true, a conviction that you accept—it doesn't have to be realistic or even technically accurate—in contrast with a thought that actively creates images or forms words in your brain.

One of the most effective beliefs on aging is the "use it or lose it" mentality concerning exercise. Gerontologists have for over twenty years demonstrated that regular physical activity throughout life (even into the late seventies) retards the loss of muscle tissue and bone commonly observed with advancing years.

Researchers at Tufts University in Boston tested this hypothesis by incorporating a weight training regimen for a group of the frailest residents in a local nursing home. The results were an astounding 300 percent increase in muscle tissue within two months. In addition, the participants' balance and coordination improved and a notable resurgence in their love of life was evident. The age range of this remarkable group was from 87 to 96.[8]

Another example of belief affecting aging characteristics comes from Lourdes in France. In Lourdes, France, in 1858, a young woman named Bernadette Soubirous received a vision of the Virgin Mary. Later a shrine was constructed there which attracted visitors with various medical problems. The belief is that bathing in the cold waters of this region will cure just about everything.

---

8   K. Dychtwald, *Age Wave* (Los Angeles: Jeremy P. Tarcher, 1989).

A Medical Bureau was established by the Catholic Church in 1883 to authenticate and study these cures. In 1954 an International Medical Committee was set up, with several medical researchers and physicians to carry on this work.

The beliefs of Nobel Laureate in Medicine Alexis Carrel changed after his first visit to the Lourdes shrine in 1903. At first he was quite skeptical about the claims being made concerning "cures" at Lourdes. As a medical director of the Rockefeller Institute, he had previous experience with exaggerated claims of healing.

Carrel studied a woman with tubercular peritonitis and was absolutely amazed at what he observed. A large, pus-filled abdominal tumor at her navel seemed to disappear within a matter of minutes of her immersion into the waters of Lourdes. This was witnessed by Carrel, who at first thought he was "suffering a hallucination."

This woman now was free of all pain, and when Carrel visited her at a local hospital later that same day her eyes were gleaming, her cheeks were rosy, and, most important of all, her abdomen was normal—with no trace of the tumor Carrel had observed just hours before. Carrel changed his beliefs about the potential of consciousness in eliciting medical cures.

Another example of this power of belief documented by the International Medical Committee of Lourdes involved Francis Pascal.[9] He wanted to believe in the Lourdes ability to cure. Pascal developed meningitis at the age of three, becoming blind and partially paralyzed as a result. Pascal's parents brought the four-year-old boy to Lourdes in August of 1938 and bathed him twice in its waters. Francis was instantly cured. After a careful review of the records, the Bureau members and additional medical experts affirmed that Pascal's paralysis and blindness were truly organic (medical). Pascal's cure was officially authenticated as a miracle by the Archbishop of Aix-en-Provence in 1949. Never underestimate the power of beliefs.

---

9   Alexis Carrel, *Voyage to Lourdes* (New York: Harper, 1950).

Every year more than three million people make a pilgrimage to Lourdes to bathe in and drink its curing waters. Over one-half million of these visitors believe in the curing powers of Lourdes and are seeking a resolution to some "medical" problem. More than sixty cures have been proclaimed as miraculous by the Catholic Church since 1858.

Such disorders as multiple sclerosis, anterolateral spinal sclerosis (ALS), tumors of the leg and abdomen, sarcoma of the pelvis, spondylitis, gangrene, and many others have been cured at Lourdes. No doubt praying at the Lourdes shrine, attending various ceremonies, and the ritual of making this pilgrimage itself all contributed to the belief mechanism in eliciting the cures at Lourdes. We can learn quite a bit about our mind-body relationship with examples such as Lourdes to apply the technique presented in part II.

The Tufts University study and the miraculous case of Francis Pascal at Lourdes illustrate the power of beliefs. When beliefs change, the body responds accordingly. This is how aging can be slowed down and actually reversed. To be empowered is to rid yourself of fear. Can you imagine what would have happened if the 87- to 96-year-old men in the Tufts study exhibited any intense fear of getting a heart attack while lifting weights?

Another classic example of the power of beliefs relates to the use of placebos in medicine. The placebo has no additives to give it any chemical activity. Yet study after study shows that about one-third of people given this placebo expecting it to work are helped by it. David Sobel, the placebo expert, says, "the placebo makes a statement that we have within us a certain self-regulatory mechanism, a self-healing mechanism, which can be mobilized given proper situational and environmental cues."[10] This also works in regard to aging.

Unquestionably, some of the best examples of beliefs in relationship to healing are found in the New Testament's references to miracles performed by Jesus. In these accounts, the faith or belief of the person

---

10 Ornstein and Sobel, op cit.

receiving healing was noted. My book *Soul Healing* discusses these biblical occurences in greater detail.[11]

Remember the difference between thoughts and beliefs described earlier. You just can't think aging away, but you may apply the mechanism of a change in your beliefs. This alteration in previous paradigms will cause the immune system to respond positively. At the same time your mind-body interaction is oblivious to conscious control. Now your defense mechanisms (the part of your conscious mind that resists change) cannot exert its usual domination over your thoughts and beliefs, resulting in a delayed aging process and increased longevity.

Now let us consider some updated consciousness-modified statements concerning aging:

- It is the diseases commonly associated with the elderly (heart disease, arthritis, cancer, and so on) that cause the physical and mental anguish observed in aging. These diseases are preventable, and aging itself is not painful.

- There is no typical aging that applies to everyone. Many avoid the classical aging symptoms (and so can you), while others exhibit diseases of aging well before their advanced years.

- Components of our body really don't age. DNA is constantly being replaced by identical new DNA. Minerals, water, and blood are also continually being renewed. These components constitute over 70 percent of our body. Our consciousness, intelligence, and personality per se do not age in the same way as matter. Certain single-celled organisms like the amoeba never age at all.

- The real cause of death is not aging but the diseases commonly associated with aging.

- A healthy lifestyle is far more important in extending your longevity than being the child of long-living parents. You will

---

11 Bruce Goldberg, *Soul Healing* (St. Paul: Llewellyn Publications, 1996).

only add about three years to your life expectancy if your parents lived to be over eighty.

- Our body's hormones (DHEA) can be adjusted through consciousness techniques (hypnosis and meditation) to greatly slow down and even reverse the aging process.

- It is quite possible, using the techniques recommended in this book, to extend your longevity to 120 years or longer living a high-quality life free of "diseases of aging."

Psychological Factors

Psychosocial factors are used by gerontologists to predict longevity. First let us consider some of these factors or circumstances that accelerate aging and shorten our lifespan:

- Excessive worry.

- Job dissatisfaction.

- Regret for sacrifices made in the past.

- Depression.

- Lack of regular work routine.

- Financial burdens.

- Getting angry easily, or being unable to express anger.

- Criticism of self and others.

- Having to work more than 40 hours per week.

- Lack of regular daily routine.

- Feeling helpless to change oneself and others.

- Loneliness, absence of close friends.

- Living alone

Contrast those circumstances with the following factors that will help extend our longevity and slow down the aging process:

- Regular work routine.

- Feeling financially secure, living within means.

- Job satisfaction.

- Happy marriage.

- Ability to laugh easily.

- Optimistic about the future.

- Regular daily routine.

- Taking at least one week's vacation every year.

- Feeling in control of personal life.

- Feeling of personal happiness.

- Ability to express feelings easily.

- Satisfactory sex life.

- Ability to make and keep close friends.

- Enjoyable leisure time, satisfying hobbies.

From these various psychosocial factors the most significant ones appear to be having a regular work schedule and daily routine. The most reliable indicator for being at risk for a heart attack is lack of job satisfaction.

The younger you are when you incorporate the principles and techniques presented in this book, the more you will benefit. The fact that the aging process is actually learned was demonstrated by a classic study conducted by Harvard psychologist George Vaillant, one of the earliest researchers to link chronic illness, premature aging, and early death with depression.

Vaillant studied 185 young men who were Harvard students during World War II. He monitored their health during the next 40 years. Those that reacted poorly to stress became depressed and were more likely to die at a young age. Only two of the subjects who demonstrated sound mental health became chronically ill or died by the age of 53. Eighteen out of the 48 men who exhibited depression were chronically ill or died by age 53. This was nine times the rate found in the men in good mental health.[12]

Dr. Vaillant's results showed that poor mental health accelerates aging and good mental health slows it down. The critical years were between 21 and 46. This period of time is when one generally fails or succeeds in establishing a level of empowerment of self. It didn't matter whether these men were the victims of abuse or other traumas during their childhood. Giving up our inner adaptability to stress makes us far more susceptible to diseases of aging than does the stress itself.

There really is no such thing as stress; it is merely our subjective interpretation of an event or thought that results in the hormonal and other physiological changes in our body that we associate with stress. For example, I am the proud owner of two miniature schnauzers (Phoenix and Alpha). I love animals and they reciprocate their feelings toward me. Let us assume I was walking down the street with someone who doesn't care for animals. If one of my neighbor's dogs were to get run over right in front of us, I would feel more stressed than the non-animal-loving companion I mentioned.

Reversing the Aging Process with Awareness

By rejecting old patterns of thought and behavior through the process of awareness, we can actually reverse aging. Harvard professor Ellen Langer selected a group of people, all in good health and over 75 in 1979, to spend a week at a country resort.[13] These subjects were instructed that

12 George Vaillant, *Adaptation of Life* (Boston: Little Brown, 1977).
13 Ellen Langer, *Mindfullness* (Reading, Mass: Addison-Wesley, 1989).

they could not bring family photos, newspapers, books, or magazines dated later than 1959.

The resort was prepared to replicate life as it was twenty years earlier (1959). All of the newspapers and magazines provided were from 1959. The music and topics of conversations and all other aspects of their week in the resort were designed to reflect their lives when they were in their mid-fifties.

Dr. Langer and her team measured the biologic ages of these subjects before, during, and at the end of this week. Having these subjects perceive themselves as being 20 years younger by shifting their awareness was supposed to have a bearing on the aging process, according to Dr. Langer's hypothesis.

Each subject wore photo identification with pictures taken 20 years earlier. Each discussion focused on the events of the late 1950s. Even references to their own personal family were from the context of 1959.

When Langer compared the results of these tests to that of a control group that went on a similar week retreat but continued to live in the world of 1979, she was happily rewarded in that her hypothesis was verified. The experimental group tested out as more self-sufficient and active. They acted more like 55-year-olds than 75-year-olds. Even those subjects who were dependent on younger family members to do certain chores for them resumed these activities.

The experimental group appeared younger by an average of three years when evaluated by an impartial panel of judges. Other changes noted in the experimental group were that they exhibited better posture, their joints were more flexible, improvements were noted in their vision, hearing, muscle strength, manual dexterity, and memory.

Professor Langer attributed these youthing changes in the experimental group to the following factors:

- The emphasis on the importance of a daily routine empowered them.

- These subjects were treated as if they actually were twenty years younger and shown respect.

- The men were asked to change their awareness and act as if they were twenty years younger.

By stimulating the consciousness of these men through a shift in awareness, Dr. Langer was able to remove 20 years psychologically from their being. The physical body simply followed suit.

The Life Force

We cannot do justice to a discussion of the effects of consciousness on aging without mentioning the concept of "life energy" or "life force." The ancient East Indian Rishis used the term *prana* to describe this life force. Prana means the basic form of energy that flows directly from pure awareness (spirit) to carry with it intelligence and consciousness to every aspect of life. This includes every physical and mental event we perceive.

The Chinese use the term *Chi* to describe this life force and control its flow through meditation, Tai Chi, and acupuncture. Other societies give this same force different names, but the principle is always the same. The more prana you possess, the more vital your bodily and mental processes. Balancing your prana is a key to a long and happy life. Some characteristics of a balanced prana are:

- Enthusiasm.
- Strong immunity.
- Proper formation of tissues.
- Physical vitality.
- Good motor coordination.
- Mental alertness.
- Balanced bodily rhythms.
- Sound sleep.

- Sense of exhilaration.

- Spiritual realization.

Aging and death result from a depleted prana. Prana is absolutely necessary to life, according to Eastern tradition. Examples of experiencing this prana are a sudden alertness, feeling overflowed with physical energy, receiving insights, and being "in the flow." Reports of a buzzing energy or streaming energy have been made of this phenomenon.

There are some simple principles to live by that will guide your consciousness to slow down the aging process. Some of these are:

- Eliminate the tendency to judge yourself and others.

- Do not seek external approval.

- Live life in the current moment and appreciate it fully. Let go of the past and do not worry about the future.

- Let go of all anger. When you do this you will facilitate your own healing moderation of aging.

- Be love-motivated rather than fear-motivated.

- Be at one with the infinite scheme of things. Practice hypnosis and meditation to attain this goal.

- Eliminate negative foods, drink, drugs, and toxic emotions from your life.

- Pay attention to your intuition and spiritual insights.

- Remember that everyone you meet, whether the meeting is a positive or negative experience, is merely a projection of your consciousness. It is what you most dislike that you most deny in yourself. What you most desire is what you most wish for in yourself. Use this to guide your spiritual growth.

- Be empowered.

You are largely responsible for your own health throughout your whole life, even well into old age.

PART II

YOUTHING —
NATURALLY

To be worthy of longevity
we must learn to be truly human
...transcending ourselves...
and not repeating history's errors.

AGING INDICATORS YOU CAN CHANGE

I call the process of slowing down (and in some cases reversing) the aging process "youthing." You may have read in other books about various drugs and supplements to combat aging, but I do not recommend these methods.

Pablo Picasso was still painting at the age of 92.

The various orthomolecular substances, drugs (including antioxidants) and vitamins that are promoted are simply not necessary. The VLC (very low calorie) diet plan in chapter 10 includes a discussion of a micronutrient-supplement plan. This particular diet reduces your daily caloric intake by 40 percent; this is the only instance where I have recommended something that is not natural.

The Spanish explorer Ponce de Leon (1460–1521) attempted to discover the "Fountain of Youth," waters which, according to legend, would transform into a young person anyone who bathed in them. This magical place was said to be surrounded by sweet-smelling flowers and huge trees bearing a rich fruit. Beautiful maidens were reported to pick the fruit for visitors.

Ponce de Leon was an old man and very anxious to find the fountain that would make him young again. He explored the islands of the Bahamas, bathing in every waterfall or stream that he found, but to no avail. When he landed in Florida, on Easter Sunday in 1513, the land was so beautiful that he was certain the Fountain was nearby. While he did not find the Fountain of Youth, he discovered Florida and claimed it for Spain.

I cannot promise you the discovery of a state, or maidens to pick fruit for you, but I can promise you longevity if you follow the recommendations in this section.

Biological Markers of Age

The focus of this book is not on merely attempting to postpone death. My intent is to show you how to maintain optimal health for the longest possible period of time.

Biomarker is a term often used to describe biological indicators of age. Researchers at the USDA Human Nutrition Research Center of Aging (HNRCA) at Tufts University in Boston have identified ten biomarkers of vitality that are possible for you to alter:

Biomarker 1: Your Muscle Mass

Biomarker 2: Your Strength

Biomarker 3: Your Basal Metabolic Rate (BMR)

Biomarker 4: Your Body Fat Percentage

Biomarker 5: Your Aerobic Capacity

Biomarker 6: Your Body's Blood-Sugar Tolerance

Biomarker 7: Your Cholesterol/HDL Ratio

Biomarker 8: Your Blood Pressure

Biomarker 9: Your Bone Density

Biomarker 10: Your Body's Ability to Regulate Its Internal
     Temperature

Biomarker 1: Your Muscle Mass

Research has demonstrated that about 6.6 pounds of lean-body mass are lost each decade of life from young adulthood to middle age. This rate accelerates after age 45. Weight lifting is an effective way to replace this lost muscle mass. We will discuss that in chapter 11.

Biomarker 2: Your Strength

Your muscles are made up of individual cells. No study has ever shown that it is possible to increase the total number of muscle cells that you have. From age 20 to about 70, we lose almost 30 percent of our total number of muscle cells. With age, the muscle cells that remain start to atrophy. Each individual cell gets smaller. The result is decreased muscular strength.[1]

Other age-related changes in your body accompany gradual muscle loss. These are:

- A declining aerobic capacity.

- A reduced blood-sugar tolerance.

- A continuing loss in bone density.

- A slowdown in your metabolism.

- A steady increase in body fat.

The good news is that a decline in muscle strength is not inevitable. Muscle mass and strength can be regained, no matter what your age and no matter what the state of your body's musculature before you start your exercise program.[2] The regimen presented in chapter 11 will assist you in this effort.

---

1 L. Larsson, G. Grimby, and J. Karlsson, "Muscle Strength and Speed of Movement in Relation to Age and Muscle Morphology," *Journal of Applied Physiology* 46(1979): 451–56.

2 W. R. Frontera, et al, "Strength Conditioning in Older Men: Skeletal Muscle Hypertrophy and Improved Function," *Journal of Applied Physiology* 64(1988): 1038–44.

Biomarker 3: Your Basal Metabolic Rate (BMR)

Your basal metabolism is the rate of your body chemistry when you are at rest. Metabolism's function is to convert food calories into energy in the form of work or heat.

Your basal metabolic rate (BMR)—or caloric expenditure at rest—declines with age. If you have a reduced amount of muscle, as most middle-aged people do, your metabolic demand for oxygen during rest declines, as does your caloric need. Older people's reduced muscle mass is almost wholly responsible for the gradual reduction of their basal metabolic rate. A person's basal metabolism drops about 2 percent per decade, starting at age 20.

Middle-aged individuals, who need fewer and fewer calories as they get older, continue eating as if they were still 20 years old. Too many calories coupled with too little exertion, a reduced musculature, and a declining metabolic rate add up to more and more fat.[3]

Biomarker 4: Your Body Fat Percentage

The average sedentary 65-year-old woman's body is about 43 percent fat tissue. Her 25-year-old counterpart's fat percentage is 25 percent. For men the body fat percentage is about 18 percent at age 25 and 38 percent by age 65. Most people assume merely losing weight is the answer to this problem. This is incorrect. Shedding fat and gaining muscle is even more important than just losing weight.

As important a factor in predicting disease as the percentage of total body mass is the distribution of body fat. People who store much of their body fat above their hips have a higher risk of developing heart disease, stroke, and diabetes than people who store fat below their hips. Even if you're not overweight, if most of your fat is stored around your waist you have a greater risk of developing one of these diseases.[4]

---

3   R. P. Donahue, R. D. Abbott, E. Bloom, et al, "Central Obesity and Coronary Heart Disease in Men," *Lancet* 8537(1987): 821–24.

4   R. E. Ostlund, Jr., et al, "The Ratio of Waist-to-Hip Circumference, Plasma Insulin Level, and Glucose Intolerance as Independent Predictors of the HDL (sub 2) Cholesterol Level in Older Adults," *New England Journal of Medicine* 322(1990): 229–34.

To maintain a more youthful-looking body we need to incorporate exercise into our regimen. The best method yet devised to lose weight without compromising our health is a combination of exercise and moderate caloric restriction. Older people, women especially, have the greatest difficulty in losing weight.

The temptation to try to lose weight by dieting alone, combined with a lower metabolic rate, only adds to this difficulty. When dieting alone is initiated fat will be lost, but so will muscle mass. A very low-calorie diet can also cause deficiencies in a whole host of nutrients, ranging from protein to vitamins and minerals. This self-starving process results in a further lowering of the BMR, which is counterproductive since the higher the BMR the faster fat is burned off.

So the solution is to include exercise with any diet plan. Here are some benefits you will gain by incorporating into your youthing regimen the exercises recommended in chapter 11:

- Raising your metabolic rate and speeding up the fat-burning process.

- Maintaining muscle mass and losing fat tissue.

- Expending more calories than you take in, because exercise consumes extra calories. You will avoid nutritional deficiencies because you will not have to radically restrict your diet. In addition, vitamin and mineral supplements are not needed.[5]

Biomarker 5: Your Aerobic Capacity

The ability to process oxygen within a given time is known as aerobic capacity. It also means effectively transporting oxygen to all parts of your body through the hemoglobin in your blood. Aerobic capacity declines with age in most people. Maximum oxygen intake begins to decline at about 20 years of age in men. In women, the decline is often postponed until the early 30s, but in both sexes, by age 65, aerobic

---

5 D. M. Seals, et al, "Endurance Training in Older Men and Women, 1: Cardiovascular Responses to Exercise," *Journal of Applied Physiology* 57(1984): 1024–29.

capacity is typically 30 to 40 percent smaller than in young adults. The decline is less in older people who exercise regularly.

Inactivity reduces the oxidative capacity of muscle cells. This explains the extreme muscular fatigue that many aging people experience. Regular aerobic exercise can bring about a large increase in the muscles' oxidative capacity, especially in older people. When older men and women do aerobic exercises, their muscle cells—not their heart or cardiovascular cells—are changed by the exertion. They build muscle mass. When older people have more muscle, they also have higher aerobic capacity because they have more muscle cells to consume oxygen.

Biomarker 6: Your Body's Blood-Sugar Tolerance

"Glucose tolerance" refers to the ability of our bodies to control blood sugar (glucose). This mechanism declines with age, making us more prone to developing "maturity-onset diabetes" (Type II diabetes). By increasing our muscle mass and lowering our body fat ratio, we can prevent this from occurring.

Maturing people who want to keep their body fat/muscle mass ratio in check and avoid diabetes should eat much less dietary fat and more fibrous carbohydrate, such as raw vegetables and whole grains. All the while, you should be doing strength-building exercises, such as weight lifting, to increase the capacity of your muscles. Strength-building exercise is a key to regulating your glucose metabolism.[6]

Biomarker 7: Your Cholesterol/HDL Ratio

Cholesterol is a fatty substance that is necessary for our body's functioning and plays an essential role in the construction of cell membranes and the production of certain sex hormones. Proteins are aligned with cholesterol (and called lipoproteins) as they circulate through our bloodstream. *Atherosclerosis* is a term applied to deposits of cholesterol,

---

6   J. W. Anderson and N. J. Gustafsson, "Type II Diabetes: Current Nutrition Management Concepts," *Geriatrics* 41(1986): 28–38.

called plaque, that lodge in tissues. This can cause heart disease and other circulatory problems.

Our blood contains four major classes of lipoproteins. These are: chylomicrons, very-low-density lipoproteins (VLDLs), low-density lipoproteins (LDLs), and high-density lipoproteins (HDLS).

The problem types of cholesterol are the LDL and VLDL, which cause plaque deposits to form in the coronary arteries. HDL cholesterol counteracts this by cleansing the arteries of plaque and actually functioning to prevent heart disease.

Physicians recommend periodic cholesterol counts to check the status of your blood's cholesterol. If your total cholesterol level is under 200, that is good, but don't assume that you have no blood chemistry risk of heart disease. You must raise the HDL cholesterol and lower the LDL cholesterol in your blood to protect yourself against heart disease.

A cholesterol count looks like this:

$$\frac{\text{Total Cholesterol}}{\text{HDL Cholesterol}} = \text{Your Cholesterol/HDL Ratio}$$

The total cholesterol/HDL ratio goal for middle-aged and older men should be 4.5 or lower. For women, this ratio needs to be 3.6 or less.[7]

As we age, the harmful LDL and VLDL classes of cholesterol increase. A combination of regular physical activity and a reduction in saturated fat and cholesterol (egg yolk, for example) from our diet will raise good HDL and lower harmful LDL cholesterol levels, but diet alone will not raise the HDL cholesterol levels. The best combination is diet, exercise, quitting smoking, and going off birth-control pills.[8] Other medications that cause cholesterol problems are anabolic steroids and diuretics. I will further discuss cholesterol in chapter 10.

---

7   N. F. Gordon and L. W. Gibbons, *The Cooper Clinic Cardiac Rehabilitation Program* (New York: Simon & Schuster, 1990), p. 195.

8   D. Streja and D. Mymim, "Moderate Exercise and High-Density Lipoprotein Cholesterol," *Journal of the American Medical Association* 243 (1979): 2190–2192. See also M. M. Dehn and C. B. Mullins, "Physiologic Effects and Importance of Exercise in Patients with Coronary Artery Disease," *Cardiovascular Medicine* 4 (April 1977): 31–47.

Biomarker 8: Your Blood Pressure

Hypertension (high blood pressure) is often called the "silent killer" because it doesn't exhibit clinical symptoms. Over 60 million Americans have hypertension. This disorder can cause heart attacks, strokes, and other life-threatening diseases.

The following factors may bring on hypertension: too little exercise, obesity, too much salt and fat in the diet, alcohol, and smoking

Race is also a factor with hypertension. Blacks are far more prone to age-related high blood pressure than whites. A large number of communities and populations around the world show no increase in blood pressure with age.[9] Unfortunately, America is not one of them. Normal blood pressure is less than 140 systolic and less than 85 diastolic. To illustrate the significance of exercise in reducing blood pressure, scientists at Dallas' Cooper Clinic Institute for Aerobics Research found that people who maintain their fitness have a 34 percent lower risk of developing hypertension (see footnote 7).

Biomarker 9: Your Bone Density

As we age the mineral content of our bones declines, leaving older people with a weaker and more brittle skeleton. Here again there is a race differential; Asians and Caucasians are more at risk than black people. Osteoporosis is a term applied to a mineral loss to the extent that there is a great risk of bone fracture. This factor is neither necessary nor a normal component of aging.

Broken bones are the leading cause of accidental death in the frail elderly. Fractures of the hipbone are particularly lethal. Our bones are in a dynamic state. We are continually forming bone (calcification) and reshaping it (resorption).

Since stress placed on a bone repeatedly causes it to get stronger rather than weakening it, weight-bearing exercises (such as walking, running, and cycling), continued over an 8-to-24-month time span,

---

9 A. S. Truswell, B. M. Kehnelly, J. D. L. Hansen, and R. B. Lee, "Blood Pressure of Kung Bushmen in Northern Botswana," *American Heart Journal* 84 (1972): 5–11.

can effectively reduce the rate of bone loss. This is true even in the most at-risk population, postmenopausal women.[10]

An individual experiences approximately one percent loss of bone mass per year. Research shows that two weeks of complete bed rest can cause as much calcium loss from bones as one whole year's worth of aging. Exercise may help foster the body's calcium absorption from the blood and the formation of new bone to reduce this bone loss.

Biomarker 10: Your Body's Ability to Regulate Its Internal Temperature

Our body has a natural mechanism that maintains its temperature within a degree of 98.6 Fahrenheit or 37.5 centigrade. The elderly suffer from dehydration and heart-related injuries because the body's vital thermoregulatory ability diminishes with age. In general, older people don't drink enough water.[11] Even when they exert themselves in the heat, often they still fail to replenish their body's water stores in sufficient quantities.

In addition, it takes a warmer internal temperature to make an older kidney function. An impaired ability to concentrate urine also has a lot to do with older people's dehydration and thermoregulatory problems. The older you are, the more fluids you must force yourself to drink even when you're not thirsty.

Regardless of your age, if your body is in shape you will:

- Sweat more when you work out in the heat. Sweating is the body's primary way of cooling itself.

- Have higher total body water content. Regular exercise increases the amount of water in your blood.

- Lose fewer "electrolytes." (potassium, sodium, and chloride).

---

10 B. Dawson-Hughes, P. F. Jacques, and C. N. Shipp, "Dietary Calcium Intake and Bone Loss from the Spine in Healthy Postmenopausal Women," *American Journal of Clinical Nutrition* 46 (1987): 68–87.

11 P. A. Phillips et al, "Reduced Thirst After Water Deprivation in Healthy Elderly Men," *New England Journal of Medicine* 311 (1984): 753–59.

Erdman Palmore of Duke University studied aging on 268 subjects and listed the following factors as the best predictors of longevity:

- Each person's actuarial life expectancy.

- Physical health.

- Work satisfaction.

- Scores on intelligence tests.

Palmore stated, "The most important overall factors in longevity among the aged are health maintenance (especially avoiding cigarettes); and maintaining a useful and satisfying role and positive view of life."[12]

Lester Breslow and Norman Breslow studied 7,000 residents of Alameda County, California, in the San Francisco Bay Area. Their findings revealed that no smoking, weight within 20 percent of that recommended for one's age, sex, and height; moderate alcohol intake; moderate exercise about three times a week; regular meals, including breakfast; and sleeping seven or eight hours a night were effective guidelines for enjoying a longer life.

A most startling observation they made was that 70-year-olds who followed all these health rules were as healthy as people aged 35 to 44 who practiced only three of the rules. This antiaging regimen was responsible for the male study participants living, on average, an extra eleven years and the females living an extra seven.[13]

Isn't Aging Just Genetic?

I was trained to assume aging was almost entirely genetic. Having degrees in biology, chemistry, dentistry, and counseling psychology, I felt the scientific paradigms were reasonably well developed.

---

12 Erdman Palmore, "Predicting Longevity: A New Method," *Normal Aging II: Reports from the Duke Longitudinal Study, 1970–1973* (Durham, North Car.: Duke University Press, 1974).

13 Lester Breslow, "Health Priorities and Quality Care Evidence from Alameda County" *Preventive Medicine: An International Journal Devoted to Prace and Theory,* January 1993.

Studies with identical twins acted to buttress this conclusion. Identical twins develop when a fertilized egg divides in two before attaching to the uterine wall and commencing normal growth. The resulting pair of eggs contain the exact same genetic makeup. Even if these twins were separated at birth and had no contact with each other in different environments, according to the genetic aging theory their aging should be very similar.

Jim Lewis and Jim Springer were identical twins separated four weeks after birth and adopted by different Ohio couples. Many years later they were reunited and showed astonishing similarities. Their respective adopted parents gave them the same first name, both drove Chevys and chewed their fingernails, each named his dog Toy and married a woman named Linda, divorced her and then married a woman named Betty. In addition, both had worked as gas-station attendants and sheriff's deputies, and in each of their gardens stood a tree encircled by a white wooden bench.[14]

This case study would seem to give tremendous weight to genes controlling our aging. However, the work conducted by Danish psychiatrist Niels Juel-Nielsen beginning in the 1950s places this conclusion in a much different light.

This researcher intimately studied twelve sets of twins by interviewing them and taking their personal and medical histories, along with psychiatric and medical tests. Twenty years later, when most of them had reached old age, he repeated this procedure.[15]

Kamma and Ella, separated the day after they were born, both grew up in rural Denmark. When Juel-Nielsen first met them, in their middle age, "it was difficult to specify how they differed." Both were calm, initially reserved, but later more talkative. Both were of average intelligence, wore glasses and had developed migraine headaches when they were about 10.

---

14 A. Leaf, "The Aging Process: Lessons from Observations in Men," *Nutrition Review* (February 1988): 8.
15 Ibid.

Kamma developed heart problems at 50 and survived a heart attack at age 59. She had a second heart attack the following year, was diagnosed with breast cancer at 68, had a mastectomy and died soon after from a massive internal hemorrhage. Ella, on the other hand, had a mild case of diabetes, slight hypertension, and was alive and well at age 73. She was in fairly good health and had never been hospitalized.

"Like my predecessors," Juel-Nielson wrote, "I never reached any general conclusion or definitive solution to the nature-nurture problem." Similar conclusions, or lack of certainty, have been drawn by modern researchers James Fozard, Ph.D., director of the National Institute on Aging's Baltimore Longitudinal Study on Aging, psychiatrist John Brettner of the Duke University Medical Center, Thomas Bouchard, Jr., Ph.D., and James Vaupel, Ph.D., of the University of Minnesota, Sandra Scarr, Ph.D., of the University of Virginia and psychiatrist Lissy Jarvik of the UCLA Neuropsychiatric Institute.

Twin studies may debunk the idea that a genetic switch sets a maximum limit on our life span. The ways they may come to differ in later years, then, must be due to environmental influences. Our lifestyle does affect the aging process. If you come from a family with poor genes, don't give up. The next five chapters will show you what you can do to look younger and live longer naturally.

SIMPLE, NATURAL METHODS TO LOOK YOUNGER

There are many things we can do to keep our skin from showing signs of aging, but paramount among them is avoiding the sun. Sunlight and heat damage the skin's collagen and elastic fibers. Wrinkles develop when our facial movements repeatedly fold skin that's no longer as elastic as it was.

At 89, Mary Baker Eddy was directing the Christian Science Church.

Other environmental conditions contribute to aging skin: harsh soap, wind, cold, or any traumas felt by the skin.

Keeping Your Skin Young

To maintain your skin health you should avoid harsh cleaners and astringents, use a mild soap, and apply a moisturizer after washing to help counter dryness. The following washing regimen is very good for your skin:

Step 1: Start with a cleansing lotion. Pour about a teaspoon of it onto a washcloth. Massage into the skin using a gentle, upward motion from the center of the face to the sides. Include the neck, also using upward strokes. Rinse thoroughly with warm water.

Step 2: If you enjoy using soap, follow Step 1 with your usual washing. Be sure to use a mild, nonalkaline brand that will not
destroy the skin's delicate acid balance.

Step 3: Saturate a cotton ball with a mild skin freshener made of
equal parts of witch hazel and cucumber juice. Dab gently on
the skin.

Step 4: Splash with cold water to rinse off any remaining freshener
and to close the pores and stimulate the circulation.

Step 5: Gently pat dry with a towel. Then, when the skin is dry, apply
a light moisturizer. This step is important because it helps the skin
retain moisture while protecting it from dirt and pollution.

Most people show the following skin changes as they age:

- Your skin turns from a rosy color to a more yellowish hue.

- Your skin gets rougher and less evenly pigmented (age spots).

- You lose 50 percent of the Langerhans cells, the immune cells
that protect against skin cancer.

- You lose 10 percent to 20 percent of your skin's pigment cells
each decade.

- You lose elasticity.

Liver spots are flat brown spots that emerge about the time we reach
our fifties. The spots are caused by the sun and have nothing to do with
the liver. By applying lemon juice daily you can lighten them somewhat. Stay out of the sun as much as possible, or at least use a protec-
tive sunscreen. Most brands are labeled with a number from 2 to 15.
The higher the number, the greater the protection.

Diet can be helpful in maintaining a youthful glow to the skin. The
following chart will assist you in choosing a balanced diet to prevent
vitamin and mineral deficiencies and their associated negative effect on
the skin:

Nutrient	Effect on Skin	Food Source
vitamin A	deficiency leads to dry, scaly rough skin	leafy green vegetables, carrots, apricots, peaches
vitamin C	prevents easy bruising of capillaries and blotchiness	green peppers, guavas, papayas, citrus fruits, tomatoes
vitamin E	antioxidant; softens scar tissue	wheat germ, whole-grain bread, oatmeal, cooking oils
vitamin B2	contributes to healthy working of oil glands	yogurt, milk, broccoli
niacin	deficiency leads to rough, red skin	liver, beef
vitamin B6	deficiency leads to excessively oily skin	wheat germ, bran, eggs, liver
EFAs	essential fatty acids help prevent dryness	fish, vegetable oils
iron	rich blood for maximum cell nourishment	liver, leafy green vegetables, peanuts
protein	building block of all tissue	fish, liver, meats, milk, legumes
zinc	deficiency leads to dry, scaly skin and impairs wound-healing	red meats, shellfish

Preventing Aging Around the Eyes

The skin around the eyes is thin and subjected to the mechanical stress of squinting and blinking. Retention of oil by this skin often results in a puffy appearance. Aging weakens the muscle tone and the loss of skin elasticity contributes to crow's feet and bags under the eyes.

These hints will assist you in your goal to retain a youthful appearance to the skin around your eyes:

- Don't smoke. It dries your skin, makes you squint (thus imprinting crow's feet), and robs your body of vitamin C.

- Get enough sleep.

- Don't rub your eyes. Rubbing stretches the thin eye skin and encourages bags.

- Use a substantial sunscreen (protection factor 15) whenever you go outside.

- Use a moisturizer—heavy on the eyelid, lighter on the under-eye—night and day.

Other suggestions that will help slow down aging of your skin are:

- Plug in a humidifier or place an open pan of water on a radiator or stove to reduce exposure to dry air. Low humidity can prematurely age skin by robbing it of natural moisture and making it prone to wrinkles.

- Take brief showers instead of baths, especially during the winter. Long, hot baths dry the skin by washing away natural oils. Use bath oils if you must take a bath.

- Avoid taking diuretics (water-reduction pills), which dry the skin from the inside out.

- Exercise regularly. This increases blood flow and bathes the skin in its natural moisturizer, sweat. Exercise may also help reduce the tension and stress that eventually etch the face with lines and creases.

Keeping Your Hair Young

Normal aging does not damage our hair. We do the damage by an improper diet, applying harsh chemicals, and other abuses. The recommendations that follow will ensure that you will have hair as lustrous and full-bodied in your 30s and 40s as you did in your 20s.

Your diet can help keep your hair looking good. Here are some nutritional recommendations:

Nutrient	Need	Source
Protein	Hair is 98 percent protein	fish, eggs, meats, cheese
B vitamins	counteract effects of stress; stimulate cell growth and repair	whole grains, eggs, liver, wheat germ
vitamin E	promotes healthy scalp	green vegetables, seeds, nuts, whole grains
vitamin C	repairs follicle injury	citrus fruits, leafy vegetables
Calcium	hair and nail strength	dairy products
Zinc	cell growth, vitamin synthesis	shellfish, red meat, wheat germ

Caring for Your Hair

Here are some classic myths about hair care, and the true facts:

- MYTH: Sun-drying is natural and good for your hair.
  FACT: The sun dries out your hair and causes split ends.

- MYTH: Split ends can be cured.
  FACT: They cannot be treated. Simply cut them off.

- MYTH: It is ideal to brush your hair 100 strokes to keep it healthy.
  FACT: Twenty gentle strokes is far better. You can cause baldness by brushing your hair too much or too vigorously.

- MYTH: Shampoos and conditioners make your hair thicker:
  FACT: Hair is dead tissue. Its structure can't be improved.

Additional hints to slow down the aging of your hair are:

- Most hair-coloring solutions, permanent-wave mixtures, hair
  straighteners, and shampoos cause chemical damage to your hair.
  Select a shampoo with a PH close to the hair's own 4.5 to 5.5.
  Use a high PH (alkaline) hair product with a low PH (acidic)
  rinse after any hair treatment.

- Try not to use hair spray. It is mostly alcohol and makes the
  hair shaft brittle and liable to breaking. A dull appearance
  may also result when the sticky film left by the spray attracts
  dust to your hair.

- Cover your hair when you are in the sun to prevent split ends.

- Avoid blow dryers. They scorch the scalp and create split ends.
  Use a low-wattage dryer, if you must, and keep it as far from
  your scalp as you can.

- Hairstyles such as ponytails, braids, and any style requiring tightly clamped barrettes or rubber bands subject the hair to excess
  tension and can cause traction baldness. It is best to avoid these
  styles, but if you must wear some type of fastener, never keep it
  in your hair overnight.

Getting Better Sleep

Insomnia is more frequent in older people. Many people past 50
require only 4½ to 6½ hours of sleep. Their sleep is also lighter. Adjust
your bedtime schedule to the amount of sleep you need to avoid toss-
ing and turning from frustration.

Sleeping difficulties may be brought about by worry, depression,
pain, the use of drugs that alleviate depression, or some other factor.
You can avoid most insomnia by eating foods rich in tryptophan, such

as eggs, meats, and certain fish—bluefish and salmon, in particular. Carbohydrates give tryptophan speedy passage to the brain. If you've been eating tryptophan-high foods during the day, try eating some whole wheat toast or a banana just before bed.

Not taking your problems to bed with you will also aid your sleep. Make an effort to go to bed at the same time each night. Refrain from napping during the day.

The following exercise while lying in bed will help you fall asleep faster:

- Tense the muscles in each part of the body starting from the feet and continuing to the head.

- Now relax each muscle. Repeat this procedure until you drop off to sleep.

A simple self-hypnosis script that will eliminate insomnia quickly is given in chapter 13.

Varicose Veins

Symptoms such as soreness, tenderness, swelling, night cramps, and the appearance of swollen, bluish cordlike veins on the legs indicate you have varicose veins. People who stand a lot, those people with parents or grandparents who had varicose veins, most women, and obese people are likely candidates for this disorder.

As we age our veins become less elastic and the supporting muscles weaker. Varicose veins result from this combination. One of the best natural treatments for this is exercise. Regular workouts will prevent you from getting varicose veins, and ease the discomfort if you already have them.

Some physicians recommend a high fiber diet. Other experts suggest going barefoot at home because it strengthens the foot muscles and improves blood flow.

A Healthier and Younger Back

Your mattress is most likely the cause of your back problems. A too soft or too hard mattress will aggravate this situation, but a hard orthopedic bed is still the first choice, especially for low-back pain sufferers, according to a study conducted by researchers at the division of orthopedics and rehabilitation, University of California at San Diego. Waterbeds are an acceptable alternative.

When you shop for a mattress, consider the following hints. When trying out a mattress, you need to lie on it for at least ten minutes to get the real feel of it. Don't rely on a label such as "super-firm" or "ortho-firm," no matter how medically impressive it may sound; there are no industry-wide standards.

As for sleeping positions, a straight spine imposes the least strain. Alternatively, if you suffer from low back pain, try sleeping like a baby—on your side, curled up in a semifetal position. For people who insist they can only sleep on their stomachs, placing a pillow under the pelvis will relieve lower back sag.

Keeping Your Teeth and Gums Young

You don't have to floss all of your teeth, just the ones you want to keep. Ignore your teeth and they will go away. Do these remarks sound familiar? When I practiced dentistry I would receive coffee mugs, pencils, and calendars from various companies with these witty little oral health reminders.

The main cause of cavities is sugar. However, sugar substitutes used in mints and gum (Xylitol, Mannitol, and Sorbitol) can also generate dental decay. Foods destructive to tooth enamel include foods rich in acid (fruits), cola drinks, and food high in phosphorus (poultry, fish, red meat, carbonated soft drinks, and flour).

You increase your risk for cavities when you repeatedly sip sugar-containing soft drinks, exposing teeth to a constant sugar bath; when you eat sticky sweets that can remain on and between tooth surfaces for a prolonged period, or when you regularly eat sugary foods between meals or that remain in your mouth for a long time.

Healthy Choices

The following foods will help maintain your oral health:

- Aged cheddar, Swiss, and Monterey Jack cheeses.

- Wheat germ, bran, peanuts and walnuts.

- Sage and garlic.

- Leafy green vegetables, fruits and other foods high in vitamin C.

- Milk, yogurt, cheese, and other foods high in calcium.

The American Dental Association suggests the following to maximize your teeth and gums:

- Use a fluoride toothpaste or gel.

- Limit foods containing sugar, especially sticky sweets and sweets (like hard candy) that linger in the mouth.

- Eat a balanced diet to help maintain the gums and bones that support your teeth.

- Remove plaque by thoroughly brushing and flossing at least once a day. Use a soft bristle brush with rounded ends and a flat brushing surface.

- Get regular checkups.

Reducing Eye Strain to Keep Your Eyes Young

This approach is based on the Chinese system of acupressure. Shut your eyes and cover them with your palms before you start the following exercises. Rest your elbows on a desk or table and relax for a minute or two, then remove your palms.

- Points around the eye socket. Make fists and place them against the eyebrows with your thumbs at the temples. Rub all around the eye sockets several times with the middle joint of the forefinger.

- Points below the eye. Hook your thumbs under your chin and place both forefingers just below the eye, along the bony ridge halfway between the nose and the far end of the eye. Rub toward the inside, then toward the outside. Repeat.

- Points on either side of the nose. Use the thumb and forefingers of either hand to press and squeeze two points on either side of your nose just below your eyes. Press down, then squeeze up. Repeat.

- Points under the eyebrows. Resting a bent forefinger and middle finger of each hand against your forehead, use your thumbs to gently press and rub two points just under the eyebrows near the bridge of the nose. Rub toward the inside several times, then the outside. Repeat.

- Always "palm" your eyes for a minute or so and end the exercise by staring off at a distant point.

To further protect the youth of your eyes here are some additional suggestions:

- Handle chemicals cautiously. Wear goggles when spraying herbicides or pesticides in the garden. Use household cleaning solutions with care.

- Protect yourself at play. Wear heavy-duty polycarbonate goggles when playing racquet sports. When you swim, wear goggles.

- If you get a foreign object or harmful substance in your eye, don't rub it. In most cases, flushing the eye with water is the best remedy. Check the instructions on the substance you were using.

- While doing close work at a computer or elsewhere, give your eyes frequent rests. At least once every two hours, close them for a few minutes, then focus on a faraway object.

- Use safety goggles whenever you work with tools like saws, drills, chisels, and electric clippers that can scatter debris.

- Don't rely on fluorescent overhead lights when you're doing detail work or close reading. Use a tabletop lamp with a regular bulb.

- Never look directly into the sun or at ultraviolet lamps. Wear polarized, mirrored, or ultraviolet-absorbing lenses, especially when you're on the water, at the beach, or on the ski slopes.

- Get enough sleep.

Follow the chart below for nutritional recommendations for maintaining your eyesight:

Nutrient	Food Source
Vitamin A	Orange, yellow and dark green vegetables, milk, and eggs.
Zinc	Whole-grain products, wheat bran, wheat germ, meat, and seafood.
Vitamin C	Fresh fruits and vegetables
Vitamin E	Whole-grain cereals, eggs, vegetable oils, leafy greens.
Folic Acid	Green and yellow vegetables.

Protecting Your Ears from Aging

Be wary of the effects of certain drugs on your ears. The following list may be of great help in this regard:

- Antibiotics like streptomycin and neomycin are known to damage parts of the ear and cause permanent hearing loss.

- Certain cancer-treatment drugs can cause permanent damage to the ears.

- Caffeine, in excessive amounts, can cause ringing in the ears (tinnitus).

- Aspirin, in large quantities (20 tablets daily), can cause temporary hearing loss.

- Alcohol, when consistently abused, can lead to hearing loss.

- Certain powerful loop diuretics can temporarily impair hearing.

- Certain local anesthetics like lidocaine and procaine hydrochloride can cause temporary hearing loss.

To protect your ears from damage caused by excessive noise, I suggest the following:

- If you live on a noisy street, consider double-paned windows or thick drapes to help muffle the din.

- If you attend live concerts, don't position yourself near any loudspeakers.

- Use an ear-protection device whenever your environment is noisy.

- If you listen to music with earphones or a portable earplug system, turn the volume down.

Nutritional advice for better and younger hearing:

- Cut down on salt and eat potassium-rich foods like salmon, chicken, and bananas.

- Vitamin B6 helps prevent sodium retention. Leafy green vegetables, whole grains, eggs, and liver are rich sources.

- Vitamin A is a necessary component of the hair cells within the inner ear. Orange, yellow and dark green vegetables, milk, and eggs are good sources.

A DIET FOR A LONGER LIFE

UCLA's Roy Walford believes that under-nutrition—a diet that provides for all our metabolic needs, but is very low in calories—can extend the maximum lifespan of humans. Walford admits, however, that the scientific studies supporting his theory have been done only with rats, mice, or other animals—not with humans.[1]

> Grandma Moses was an active artist at 100.

The various dietary regimens presented in this chapter all follow this principle—eat light, but eat right. If you err, err on the side of too little food. You will not starve or in any way compromise your nutrition or immune system by following these recommendations. The opposite is more likely.

Beta-Carotene

Vitamin A is required to maintain the health of your teeth, nails, hair, and glands. Forty percent of Americans—particularly Hispanics and blacks—do not meet their RDA (Recommended Daily Allowance) for vitamin A. Because this fat-soluble vitamin is stored in your liver and fat, it can be toxic and cause anemia and gout.

---

1 Roy Walford, *Maximum Life Span* (New York: W. W. Norton, 1983).

A better way to obtain your vitamin A naturally is with beta-carotene. Beta-carotene is an orange first-stage (precursor) form of vitamin A. Our body converts beta-carotene into the vitamin A it needs. That means you can take the beta-carotene form of vitamin A, enjoy its vital youth benefits, yet avoid the possible toxicity of regular vitamin A.

Beta-carotene is also a powerful antioxidant, as are vitamins E and C. Research at Harvard has shown that beta-carotene may prevent or slow the development of skin cancer. It fights the free radicals that cause aging in your skin and throughout your body and has even been shown to extend life expectancy in animals, from mice to men.

Foods that are a good source of beta-carotene are:

Cantaloupe	Beets	Papaya
Broccoli	Vegetable soups	Butternut squash
Milk	Carrots	Fresh tomato sauce
Kale	Pumpkins	Parsnips
Spinach	Watercress	Sweet potatoes
Dandelion	Tomatoes	Mustard
Greens	Radishes	Chicory
Collard		

My recommendation is to eat at least one 3-ounce serving of green, red, or yellow vegetables a day to obtain adequate beta-carotene.

Bone-Building Tips

If you are at risk for premature bone weakening, you will need additional boron in your diet. The single best way to get enough boron is to eat plenty of fresh fruits and vegetables.

Our bones are mainly composed of calcium, phosphorus, and a protein called collagen. Of all these components, calcium is the most important. Each day that passes without sufficient amounts of calcium in the body is another day of bone loss. We are losing a mineral we don't get enough of in the first place. Dietary surveys show that the average woman who is 45 or older consumes the bare minimum of 450 to 500 milligrams of calcium a day.

Five hundred milligrams is far below the Recommended Dietary Allowance of 800 milligrams of calcium for women and men over 19. When calcium is needed in another part of the body, a hormone ferries some calcium from our bones to our blood, nerves, muscles, or other areas. Blood, in turn, delivers new calcium back into the bones for their vital needs, so the calcium composition of our bones is constantly in flux.

According to the National Institute of Health, Americans aren't getting enough calcium. Most women over 45 now consume less than 500 mg. of the mineral each day, but NIH recommends that they get at least 1,500 mg. Younger women and teenagers should get at lest 1,000 mg. per day, while the current recommended daily allowance of 800 mg. is probably sufficient for most men.

Mineral Sources

The following list of foods will assist your body in bone building and maintenance.

Boron: Tofu, plums, peaches, grapes, raisins, apples, wine, prunes, almonds, pears, peanuts, dates, green leafy vegetables.

Calcium: dairy products, low-fat yogurt, sardines (with bones), salmon, tofu, broccoli, spinach, collard greens, sesame seeds, seaweeds (used in Japanese cooking).

Manganese: Legumes, sunflower seeds, meat, dark-green lettuce, cloves, spinach, wheat germ, and black beans.

Magnesium: Dark green vegetables, broccoli, Brussels sprouts, spinach, dark-green lettuce.

Other tips to help prevent bone aging are:

- Avoid special very low-calorie diets, especially those with incomplete nutrients (weight-loss powders, drinks, or one-item diet programs).

- Drink fewer carbonated drinks. They are acidic, which can upset your mineral balance.

- Limit the amount of concentrated animal protein you eat. A very high-protein diet causes minerals to be flushed from the body—among them bone minerals. A more balanced, lower-protein diet helps guard against mineral depletion.

- Both rhubarb and spinach contain oxalic acid, which can block mineral absorption.

- Reduce alcohol consumption to avoid flushing out minerals.

- Eat a lot of fiber, but in natural, not supplemented forms: whole grains, brown rice, oatmeal, and bulgur are better than refined wheat bran.

To Keep Your Joints Young

Add fish oils to your diet. These function as anti-inflammatory agents and combat the premature aging and pain of arthritis. These nutrients chemically change the blood and reduce the body's own chemicals that lead to painful joint tenderness, swelling, and inflammation.

Good sources of fish oils are: tuna, salmon, sardines, mackerel, sable, whitefish, bluefish, swordfish, rainbow trout, eels, herring, and squid.

For a Healthy Digestive Tract

It makes sense to eliminate foods that cause you digestive distress. Some people may have problems with gas-producing vegetables like broccoli, cauliflower, and cabbage. Others may find milk products less and less digestible. If you suffer cramps, gas, diarrhea, or constipation, think back to what you ate during the past 48 hours.

Eating a high-fiber diet is beneficial. High-fiber foods include: bran, whole grain breads and cereals, fresh fruits, and vegetables. Reduce or eliminate alcohol, caffeine, and nicotine. These commonly abused drugs are stomach and bowel irritants that may cause heartburn and indigestion.

Moderate calories. Overeating can cause stomach bloat, heartburn, and bowel distress. High-calorie diets have been linked to gallstones.

Practice good eating habits. Make mealtime relaxing. Don't eat on the run, eat while talking, or gulp hot liquids.

With these symptoms	Eliminate or reduce
Constipation	white bread, pastries and other highly processed, refined foods; antidepressants, anti-histamines, diuretics.
Stomach pain	coffee and caffeine drinks, alcohol, nicotine, aspirin, arthritis medication, asthma medication, antihypertensives, antibiotics.
Heartburn	coffee, chocolate, alcohol, onions, peppermints.
Gas, bloating, bowel distress, diarrhea	milk and milk products, saccharin-sweetened products, coffee, tea, peanuts, broccoli, cabbage, beans, garlic.

Bran is a nutrient that provides an effective and safe way of warding off constipation. Studies have shown that bran actually normalizes bowel function in diverticular disease, and can correct a number of different bowel disorders, including constipation and diarrhea. It acts as a stool softener in cases of constipation, shortening the time it takes for food to pass through the bowels and be eliminated. With diarrhea bran works in reverse, hardening the stool and lengthening the transit time.

Dennis Burkitt, M.D., a renowned researcher and fiber enthusiast, recommends adding the following to your diet: whole grain breads and cereals, nuts, dried fruit, beans, carrots, peas, and a tablespoon or two of bran.[2] Drink at least one extra glass of water a day—you need to provide the bran with plenty of moisture to absorb.

For a Healthy, Youthful Heart

The role of cholesterol in maintaining a healthy heart is so crucial that is warrants a section of its own, but since this is a chapter about diet, here are some dietary suggestions that will be beneficial for your heart:

- Drink less coffee.

- Consume fish as a main meal at least twice weekly, but avoid fried fish.

- Eat fewer eggs or eat eggs without the yolks.

- Increase your intake of complex carbohydrates (starches).

- Greatly reduce red meats and animal fats and trim off all visible fat before cooking meat.

- When you do eat fats, make sure they are monosaturated, not saturated or polyunsaturated.

- Increase your fiber intake with whole grains, fresh fruits, and fresh vegetables. You should eat fiber with every meal.

- Reduce consumption of highly refined foods, including refined sugar.

Cholesterol

There are two one-way messengers that circulate cholesterol in our body: LDL (low-density lipoprotein) transports cholesterol from the liver to the tissues and organs; HDL (high-density lipoprotein) moves cholesterol back to the liver. By increasing the HDL carrying cholesterol back to the liver and less LDL carrying it out to the blood vessels, you can halt the process that ages the heart and arteries. The single best way to do that is by balancing the ratio of saturated fat and cholesterol you eat.

---

2   D. Burkitt, et al, *Dietary Fibre, Fibre-depleted Foods and Disease* (London: Academic Press, 1985).

By lowering your LDL below 100, your body can actually start pulling deposited fats and cholesterol out of your blood vessel walls. This will actually reverse the damage accumulated by your heart. Your blood vessels will appear smoother in six months, as well as become more elastic and open. This is youthing.

Here are some very important facts about cholesterol:

- Men's Average HDL = 45 mg/dl

- Women's Average HDL = 55 mg/dl

- The higher the HDL, the lower the risk of heart disease.

- A HDL level lower than 35 mg/dl is a major risk factor for heart disease.

Some scientists and clinicians use the ratio of total cholesterol to HDL as an index of risk for heart disease. The lower the ratio, the lower the risk.

- Total cholesterol level divided by HDL for men should equal 4.5 or less.

- Total cholesterol level divided by HDL for women should equal 3.6 or less.

Your total cholesterol count should be less than 180 mg/dl if you are under 20 and below 200 mg/dl over the age of 20. A borderline high risk level is from 200–239 mg/dl. Total cholesterol counts over 240 mg/dl are considered high risk for a heart attack.

Blood cholesterol levels change over time, especially if you change your eating or exercise patterns. More than 50 percent of Americans have blood cholesterol levels high enough to be at risk for heart disease—and most of them don't know it. When you have your blood cholesterol under control, your risk of heart disease is greatly reduced.

Blood cholesterol reductions of 15 to 25 percent, achievable by diet alone in just 2 weeks, can reduce the risk of heart disease by 30 to 50 percent.

The American Heart Association recommends that no more than 10 percent of your calories should come from saturated fat. Thus, if you eat 2,000 calories a day, you should eat no more than 200 (10 percent of 2,000) calories of saturated fat.

To reduce saturated fat in your diet, substitute fish, poultry, lean meats, whole grain brands and cereals, fruits and vegetables, and dried peas and beans for foods high in fat.

Foods High in Saturated Fat	Low Saturated Fat Choices
Beef	Fruit
round steak, roast	Vegetables
porterhouse steak	Turkey breast, roasted, baked,
ground beef, lean	broiled, without skin
Whole milk	Chicken breast, roasted,
Most cheeses	baked, broiled, without skin
Hot dogs	Fish, broiled, baked, or poached
Luncheon meats (cold cuts)	Skim milk
Doughnuts	Low-fat yogurt
Cake	1% Cottage cheese
Pork	Safflower oil
chops, ham	Corn oil
sausage, bacon	Olive oil
Butter	Margarines made with
Ice cream	polyunsaturated oils
Fried potatoes	Dried peas and beans
2% Milk	Pasta, without cheese or meat
Potato chips	Rice
Nondairy coffee creamer	Popcorn, air popped
(mfrd w/coconut oil)	Whole grain breads
	without butter

Here is another chart of suggestions that will assist you in keeping your cholesterol level low:

Instead of	Try
Bacon	Canadian bacon
Frying	Baking, broiling, or steaming
Sour cream on a baked potato	Low-fat yogurt or cottage cheese
Buttering vegetables	Vegetables with herbs and lemon, lime, or orange juice.
A red meat main dish	Pasta or rice with a little meat, skinless white meat poultry, or fish for seasoning
Meat every day	Meat three times a week or less
A fast-food burger	The salad bar
Lean ground beef	Lean, trimmed round steak, white meat poultry without skin, or fish
Commercial baked goods	Home-baked treats, using polyunsaturated oils and margarine
Cream or butter sauces	Sauces using wine or low-fat broth
Nondairy coffee creamer	Nonfat milk
Chocolate	Cocoa
Butter	Tub or soft margarine
Cooking with animal fats	Cooking with vegetable oils such as sunflower, olive, or peanut oils
Whole milk	Skim or low-fat milk

Saturated fats are oils from animal products and some plants (e.g., coconut and palm) that are solid (rather than liquid) at room temperature. Examples are meat fat, lard, butter, cream, and shortening. These fats raise blood cholesterol and increase your risk of heart diseases. Polyunsaturated fats are oils from vegetable products that are liquid at room temperature, such as safflower oil, sunflower oil, and corn oil. These fats, used in moderation, lower blood cholesterol and are helpful in removing cholesterol from the body. Substituting these fats for saturated fat in the diet can reduce your risk of heart diseases. Finally, monounsaturated fats are oils from other vegetable products that also are liquid at room temperature, such as olive oil and peanut oil. Recent evidence shows that substituting these fats (in moderation) for saturated fats helps lower blood cholesterol and reduce the risk of heart disease.

Low-fat, low-cholesterol foods are also low in calories. Eating more low-fat foods will automatically cut your calorie count and help you lose weight. Taking pounds off when you're overweight lowers blood cholesterol levels. Eating low-fat items also helps you maintain your weight if it's already at a healthy level.

Fiber for a Younger Heart

Fiber assists in youthing by preventing our body from absorbing the wrong fats from foods. The Japanese eat more fiber per capita than any other country. Their death rate due to heart attacks is one seventh that of the United States. A high-fiber diet can lower triglycerides and cholesterol by one-fifth to one-third, slowing down the aging of your entire cardiac system.

The following are good sources of fiber to slow down the aging of the heart:

apples, grapes,	oats, oat bran,	pinto beans,
potatoes, squash,	barley, lentils,	navy beans,
oranges, lemons,	chick-peas,	split peas, seeds
grapefruit	black-eyed peas	

Fish for a Younger Heart

Fish contains the best fats, the Omega-3 fatty acids, among them EPA (eicosapentaenoic acid) and DHA (docosahexaenoic acid). Among their many positive effects, they:

- Make your blood platelets less sticky.

- Reduce several chemical steps that lead to arterial lesions.

- Reduce LDL levels.

- Reduce overall cholesterol.

- Reduce blood pressure.

- Minimize inflammation.

Reducing Your Blood Pressure for a Younger Heart

Controlling your blood pressure will reduce stress to your heart. One of the best ways to do this is to eliminate salt from your diet; onions, herbs, and garlic are flavorful substitutes for salt. Eliminating, or at least reducing, the alcohol you drink is also beneficial, as is eating more fiber.

Keeping Your Immune System Young

You will dramatically reduce your cancer risk by eating more fiber and less fat, by eating more mineral- and vitamin-rich fresh vegetables, and by moderating your alcohol consumption to a reasonable level.

Reducing fat will assist the phagocytes and lower the free radicals that cause cancer. This will help the immune system function more efficiently. I also suggest you eat some of the vegetables listed below at least once a week. These vegetables contain a chemical called indole that helps prevent colon cancer.

mustard greens	cabbage	rutabaga
cauliflower	turnips	Chinese cabbage
collards	broccoli	kale
Brussels sprouts	kholrabi	

The "Antiviral Cocktail"

A mixture called "egg lecithin lipids" (AL-721) was developed in Israel to fight AIDS. This cocktail made from the ingredients found in egg yolks works like a natural antiviral agent, helping to reverse the immune-system damage done by the AIDS virus.

This cocktail may work against other viruses, such as herpes and the Epstein-Barr (associated with chronic-fatigue) syndrome.

You can make your own "Antiviral Cocktail" from natural food products by following these steps:

1. Purchase from a health food store PC-55 lecithin, a high-strength soy-lecithin concentrate. (Keep refrigerated.)

2. Add 1 tablespoon of PC-55 to 1 cup of orange or other fruit juice.

3. Let mixture sit 5 minutes, then blend until well mixed.

4. Add 1 generous tablespoon of olive oil or peanut oil, and blend thoroughly for several minutes.

5. The cocktail is best taken in the morning on an empty stomach.

6. Drink this cocktail every three days and refrigerate the vegetable oil. This is not recommended if you have high cholesterol or for AIDS patients who have cancer.

For a Younger Brain

To boost mental alertness, reduce anxiety, improve memory, and stabilize moods in general, include the following in your diet:

dried beans, peas, shrimp, oysters, and most seafood	seaweed, onions, whole grains (including the bran)	green leafy vegetables, prunes, dark chocolate, seeds, nuts, fruits

These foods are rich in copper, manganese, and iodine, the brain nutrient minerals.

There are minerals (heavy metals) such as mercury, cadmium, lead, and aluminum, that may be toxic to your brain. Lead poisoning can cause mental sluggishness and even retardation. Cadmium can lead to significant memory loss and diminished mental function.

Both aluminum and cadmium are thought to be factors in Alzheimer's disease.

You can avoid memory and other mental problems by making sure you don't:

- Prepare foods from aluminum pots or use aluminum foil. Acidic foods such as tomato juice, lemonade, vinegar, and orange juice can draw the aluminum into them.

- Live close to an airport or major highway. Blood levels high in lead have been reported in Germany where traffic is congested.

- Take antacids you buy over the counter. Aluminum is one of the main ingredients.

- Live in areas with significant levels of environmental pollution.

Final Note: NIA reports have shown that one in five older people with intellectual impairment may be able to reverse the downward slide. NIA also reports that cognitive training was found to increase older people's accuracy on standard mental-function tests, so they scored as though they were "younger."

Miscellaneous Diet Tips to Slow Down Aging

- Eat zinc-rich foods.

- Eat eggplant, yogurt, and onions frequently to combat cholesterol.

- Eat apples and citrus fruit often and supplement the diet with soybean lecithin to fight cholesterol.

- Drink an extra 8-ounce glass of water each day.

- Cut down on sweet and processed foods.

- Eat lots of raw foods, whole grains, and vegetables for bulk and to prevent bowel disease.

- Eat foods rich in calcium to keep muscles working smoothly.

- Eat foods rich in vitamin B6 to increase stamina.

- Eat foods rich in iron to keep muscles functioning properly.

- Eat foods rich in the B vitamins to help eliminate tremors.

Vitamins	Food Sources
Vitamin B6	liver, herring, salmon, nuts, brown rice
Vitamin B12	meat, liver, kidney, egg yolk, fish
Folic Acid	liver and kidneys, dark-green leafy vegetables such as spinach, wheat germ, dried peas and beans
Vitamin C	black currants, sweet peppers, broccoli, citrus fruits
Vitamin D	milk, liver oils, tuna, salmon, herring, egg yolk, margarine
Vitamin E	vegetable oils, wheat germ oil, olives, peanut oil
Minerals	**Food Sources**
Calcium	milk, cheese, dairy foods, sardines
Zinc	meat, eggs, liver, seafood
Magnesium	unrefined cereals
Chromium	whole grains, leafy green vegetables

A frugal diet cannot be overemphasized. Remember those celebrated, long-lived highland folks in the Andes, in Russian Georgia, and in the Hunza region of Pakistan that we discussed in chapter 4? Though researchers have now found their life spans to have been exaggerated, these people did live—and still do in large numbers—to ripe and vigorous old ages. All the studies of these individuals emphasized their long-range adherence to frugal though nutritious diets.

Varying our diet is also important. This is because certain foods interact with one another in ways that can be potentially quite harmful. Raw legumes, such as dried beans, peas, and peanuts, can block enzymes that help digest proteins. Cabbage and Brussels sprouts can keep the thyroid gland from getting all the iodine it needs. Spinach and rhubarb contain substances that can render certain minerals and other nutrients unabsorbable. Tea and red wine can interfere with the body's use of iron and vitamin B-12. You will not have to be concerned with these and other negative food interactions if you eat a varied diet.

Height/Weight Charts

Several years ago one of my hypnotherapy patients told me something that inspired me to burn all of the height/weight charts I had ever received. This woman worked as an actuary for a major life insurance company. She informed me that I would be sent a new height/weight chart soon.

When I asked "why, has our species all of a sudden changed since the last time I was sent one of these charts?" She told me that the new charts added ten pounds to each of the heights.

This was done so that more Americans could qualify for life insurance. Recent studies revealed that the average American was forty pounds overweight, and this prompted a change in the charts. My response was that more people would die of heart disease as a result of this added weight.

My patient informed me that the premiums were adjusted (raised) to compensate for this. Apparently, you can't sell insurance policies if nobody qualifies for coverage. I responded, "that would be equivalent to me whiting out cavities (dark spots) on a patient's X-rays, instead of removing the decay and placing a filling in the tooth." My comment fell on deaf actuarial ears.

The bottom line of this story is to ignore all height/weight ratio charts. They are simply not worth the paper they are printed on.

The height, weight, and health chart that follows is an example of what I am talking about. This chart is typical of what a life insurance company sends us doctors.

Height, Weight & Health

MEN

Height		Small	Medium	Large
Feet	Inches	Frame	Frame	Frame
5	2	128-134	131-141	138-150
5	3	130-136	133-136	140-153
5	4	132-138	135-145	142-156
5	5	134-140	137-148	144-160
5	6	136-142	138-151	146-164
5	7	138-145	142-154	149-168
5	8	140-148	145-157	152-172
5	9	142-151	148-160	155-176
5	10	144-154	151-163	158-180
5	11	146-157	154-166	161-184
6	0	149-160	157-170	164-188
6	1	152-164	160-174	168-192
6	2	155-168	164-178	172-197
6	3	158-172	167-182	176-202
6	4	162-176	171-187	181-207

WOMEN

Height		Small	Medium	Large
Feet	Inches	Frame	Frame	Frame
4	10	102-111	109-121	118-131
4	11	103-113	111-123	120-134
5	0	104-115	113-126	122-137
5	1	106-118	115-129	125-140
5	2	108-121	118-132	126-143
5	3	111-124	131-135	131-147
5	4	114-127	124-138	134-151
5	5	117-130	127-141	137-155
5	6	120-133	130-144	140-159
5	7	123-136	133-147	143-163
5	8	126-139	136-150	146-167
5	9	129-142	139-153	149-170
5	10	132-145	142-156	152-173
5	11	135-148	145-159	155-176
6	0	138-151	148-162	158-179

Weights at Ages 25–29 Based on Lowest Mortality. Weight in Pounds According to Frame (with 5 lbs. Clothing for Men, 3 lbs. For Women and in 1"-Heeled Shoes).

According to this chart, my 5-feet, 6-inch height and 130-pound medium body frame would classify me as eight to twenty-one pounds underweight. Quite a range, considering that I possess more energy now than I had when I was in college thirty years ago. I am also five pounds lighter now than I was in the mid and late 1960s. Being energetic is a very important factor in eliminating "underweight" labels. Even if you fudged my body frame to the small frame category, I would still be six to twelve pounds underweight.

Below is another height/weight chart from the U.S. Center for Health Statistics, North American Association Study of Obesity:

Ideal Weight Chart

Height	Sex	Age: 18–24	25–34	35–44	45–54	55–64
4'10"	Women	114	123	133	132	135
4'11"	Women	118	126	136	136	138
5'0"	Women	121	130	139	139	142
5'1"	Women	124	133	141	143	145
5'2"	Men	130	139	146	148	147
5'2"	Women	128	136	144	146	148
5'3"	Men	135	145	149	154	151
5'3"	Women	131	139	146	150	151
5'4"	Men	139	151	155	158	156
5'4"	Women	134	142	149	153	154
5'5"	Men	143	155	159	163	160
5'5"	Women	137	146	151	157	157
5'6"	Men	148	159	164	167	165
5'6"	Women	141	149	154	160	161
5'7"	Men	152	164	169	171	170
5'7"	Women	144	152	156	164	164
5'8"	Men	157	168	174	176	174
5'8"	Women	147	155	159	168	167
5'9"	Men	162	173	178	180	178
5'10"	Men	166	177	183	185	183
5'11"	Men	171	182	188	190	187
6'0"	Men	175	186	192	194	192
6'1"	Men	180	191	197	198	197
6'2"	Men	185	196	202	204	201

According to this "ideal weight" chart I am 37 pounds underweight (being 49 years *young*). Please note that this chart makes no distinction between small, medium, and large frames. Enough said.

One important principle of physiology you should know is that 3500 calories equals one pound. The average American 150-pound male needs to consume about 2400 calories to maintain weight. The figure for women is about 2000 calories.

Dr. Walford of UCLA, to whom I referred earlier, is a great proponent of undernutrition or restricted calorie diets. Do not confuse undernutrition with malnutrition. Walford's diet of 60 percent of normal calories contains the necessary nutrients to sustain our body.

When Walford placed mice that were the equivalent of 30 to 33 human years old on this restricted diet, he observed they lived 20 percent longer than the control group. This is equivalent to 15 additional human years. These mice had a much smaller incidence of tumors and heart disease, and displayed excellent health all their lives.

We all have a metabolic set point, a mechanism in our brain that tells us when we are hungry or when we are satiated. By going against our set point our brain creates cravings for food. Walford's diet gradually altered this set point.

Dr. Walford believes his diet regimen will extend human life to 120 or older. He stated, "The idea is to lose weight gradually over the next four to six years, until you're 10 to 25 percent below your set point. That's the weight you'll drift toward if you neither overeat nor undereat. Usually it's what you weighed between ages 25 and 30."[4]

Walford's diet projection reduces the typical American's 37 percent of fat to a mere 11 percent. This alone would result in improvements in health, especially in relation to cardiovascular disease and cancer. This fat content level has been promoted by cardiologist Dean Ornish, by diet expert Pritikin, and by Duke University (where the rice diet was developed).

---

4   Walford, op cit.

When cutting calorie intake by 40 percent there simply is no room for cookies, hamburgers, French fries, cakes, and the like. We have to eliminate processed foods and empty calories from our daily diet, and this also is quite healthy.

When commenting on the greater quality of health exhibited by these underfed mice on Walford's diet, Dr. Leonard Hayflick (one of America's leading gerontologists) stated, "The restricted mice are merely being allowed to reach the limit of their life span. It's overfeeding that kills the control group."[5] Walford feels that his diet simply delays a breakdown in the immune system.

Low-Calorie Diet Slows the Aging Process

We refer to a reduced calorie diet (60% of the normal allotted calories) as a VLC (very low calorie) diet. Animal studies show that longevity increases by 50, 65, and even 83 percent (that is equivalent to a 137-year lifespan in humans). It is assumed that these dramatic results are brought about by reducing body fat, which in turn diminishes toxic free radicals, and lowers cancer and heart-disease risk.

Other advantages to a VLC diet are:

- Helps to stabilize the blood sugar imbalances in diabetes.

- Helps the body run at peak metabolic efficiency.

- Lowers cholesterol and heart-disease risk.

- Reduces muscle oxygen loss, and improves muscle function.

- Reduces free-radical damage to the body's tissues.

- Lowers blood pressure.

- Reduces destructive antibodies that attack the brain.

- Reduces the loss of certain brain cells.

---

5   Leonard Hayflick, "Recent Advances in the Cell Biology of Aging," *Mechanisms of Aging and Development*, Vol. 14 (1980).

- Strengthens the immune system.

- Slows the aging process.

There are three principles to consider in implementing a VLC diet: your diet must be more efficient, since you are eating so much less food; the plan should be incorporated correctly and gradually; and reducing calories means a longer life.

Although this plan may sound extreme, it definitely works. As a responsible doctor I must include certain precautions if you decide to undertake this VLC diet:

- Check with your physician before starting this plan.

- Eat bulk foods rich in fiber and low in calories to help you feel full. Try to eat 50 grams of fiber daily.

- Phase into this regimen gradually to prevent rapid weight loss. You may cut down to 90 percent, then 80, 70, and finally 60 percent of your normal calorie intake, over a period of several months.

- Eat smart. Eliminate refined and highly processed foods. Minimize the intake of sugar. Consume 80 grams of protein and no more than 300 grams of cholesterol daily. Fats should represent a maximum of 20 percent of your total daily calories.

Take a strong, wide-spectrum micronutrient supplement to make certain you receive all the necessary vitamins, minerals, and amino acids that are listed in the chart that follows. Please note that this is the only time in this book I recommend a supplement to your diet.

This chart comes from the U.S. Center for Health Statistics, North American Association Study of Obesity.

Vitamins		Bioflavinoids:	
Vitamin A	20,000 I.U.	Rutin	400 mg
Beta-carotene	20,000 I.U.	Hesperidin	400 mg
Vitamin B1 (thiamine)	100 mg		
Vitamin B2 (riboflavin)	100 mg	Minerals:	
Vitamin B3 (niacin)	100 mg	Calcium	400 mg
Vitamin B5	200 mg	Iron	10 mg
(pantothenic acid)		Magnesium	200 mg
Vitamin B6 (pyridoxine)	50 mg	Selenium	100 mg
Vitamin B12	200 mg	Zinc	50 mg
Vitamin C	2,000 mg		
Vitamin D	400 I.U.		
Vitamin E	200 I.U.		
Biotin	100 mcg		
Choline	200 mg		
Folic acid	400 mg		
Inositol	200 mg		

The next chart (page 130) shows recommended weight to height ratios using a very low calorie diet. This is the only chart that doesn't classify me as grossly underweight. My 49-year young body frame is only four pounds below the recommendations of this chart.

You may calculate how many calories you need to consume daily to maintain your VLC chart weight. A 50-year-old woman who is five feet seven inches, for example, would need to eat 1441 calories (131 x 11) daily; 1644 calories are required for a man the same age and height (137 x 12).

If you follow a VLC diet plan, be prepared for a surprise. A new leaner, younger, and healthier you will emerge.

VLC Height/Weight Chart

Height		18–24	25–34	Age 35–44	45–54	55–64
4'10"	Women	92	99	107	106	108
4'11"	Women	95	101	109	109	110
5'0"	Women	97	104	111	111	114
5'1"	Women	99	106	113	114	116
5'2"	Men	104	111	117	118	117
5'2"	Women	102	109	115	117	118
5'3"	Men	108	116	119	123	121
5'3"	Women	105	111	117	120	121
5'4"	Men	111	121	124	126	124
5'4"	Women	107	114	119	122	123
5'5"	Men	114	124	127	130	128
5'5"	Women	110	117	121	126	126
5'6"	Men	118	127	131	134	132
5'6"	Women	113	119	123	128	129
5'7"	Men	122	131	135	137	136
5'7"	Women	115	122	125	131	131
5'8"	Men	126	134	139	141	139
5'8"	Women	118	124	127	134	134
5'9"	Men	130	138	142	144	142
5'10"	Men	133	142	146	148	146
5'11"	Men	137	146	150	152	150
6'0"	Men	140	149	154	155	150
6'1"	Men	144	153	158	158	158
6'2"	Men	148	157	162	163	161

Sample 7-Day VLC Diet Plan

DAY 1

Breakfast:

½ grapefruit

1 poached egg

2 slices whole-wheat toast with unsweetened preserves

Lunch:

1½ cups whole-wheat pasta salad with vegetables

1 cup cabbage slaw

2 rye crackers

Dinner:

Mixed salad with oil, vinegar, and herbs

1 large baked potato

1 cup wax beans

5 ounces liver and onions

DAY 2

Breakfast:

1 cup cooked oatmeal

1 banana

1 cup skim milk

Lunch:

Tomato stuffed with chicken salad

1 whole-wheat bagel

Mixed fruit with low-fat yogurt

Dinner:

Mixed green salad with oil, vinegar, and herbs

1 cup lentil soup

1½ cups whole-wheat pasta primavera

2 pieces whole-wheat Italian bread

DAY 3

Breakfast:

1 cup puffed wheat

1 peach

1 cup skim milk

Lunch:

½ grapefruit

½ cup low-fat cottage cheese with chopped vegetables

1 whole-wheat biscuit

Dinner:

Arugula salad with oil, vinegar, and herbs

1 cup rice

5 ounces lean steak, with peppers, onions, tomatoes

1 whole-wheat roll

DAY 4

Breakfast:

1 cup Nutri-Grain™

1 banana

1 cup skim milk

Lunch:

1½ cups 3-bean salad on

bed of lettuce

1 cup chilled steamed broccoli

2 rice cakes

Dinner:

Spinach salad with low-fat, yogurt-based dressing with dill

Small butternut squash

1 cup French-cut green beans

4 ounce lamb chop

1 whole-wheat roll with 1 tsp. butter

DAY 5

Breakfast:
> 2 whole-wheat waffles topped with
> Low-fat yogurt and strawberries

Lunch:
> Taco shell, stuffed with lettuce and tomato
> ½ cup beans
> ½ cup grapes

Dinner:
> Arugula salad with oil, vinegar, and herbs
> 1 cup rice and herbs
> 1 zucchini, steamed
> 5 ounces broiled lobster tail

DAY 6

Breakfast:
> 1 cup cooked oat bran
> 1 apple
> 1 cup skim milk

Lunch:
> 1½ cups minestrone soup
> 1 slice whole-wheat toast with
> 1 ounce melted low-fat cheese
> 1 apple

Dinner:
> Arugula salad with oil, vinegar, and herbs
> 1 cup herbed barley and peapods
> 5 ounces broiled mackerel

DAY 7

Breakfast:

1 melon wedge

1 egg yolk, 2 egg whites, as omelet or scrambled

2 whole-wheat biscuits with

1 tsp. butter

Lunch:

4 oz sardines in water or tomato sauce

2 slices whole-wheat bread

Lettuce and tomato

1 orange

Dinner:

Endive salad with oil, vinegar, and herbs

1 cup zucchini and tomato

9 shrimp, sauteed in olive oil and garlic, over

1 cup rice

To use this plan correctly, be stingy in using fat or oil in cooking and serving. Be generous with your portions of salads and vegetables. This regimen is approximately 60 percent carbohydrate, 20 percent fat, and 20 percent protein. Men should increase their servings of carbohydrates and salads to provide the extra calories they need.

Final Thoughts about VLC Diet Plans

It is quite understandable that you would not want to incorporate this plan immediately, or to the extent for which it was designed. I always recommend this be gradually introduced, even if you did choose to follow it to the letter. As a "free-will activist" I empower you to make your own decisions.

For example, you may choose to only reduce your caloric intake by 20 percent, instead of 40 percent. A compromise on your height/weight ratio as indicated on the chart included is another choice for you to consider. A target weight halfway between what the chart gives and what other charts state is better than no change at all.

One thing I can guarantee is that by losing weight and reducing your caloric intake, you will look younger, feel better, have more energy, improve your health, and live longer. The choice, as always, is yours.

EXERCISE YOUR WAY TO LONGEVITY

I t is a big mistake to assume that advancing age is a static, irreversible biological condition of unwavering decrepitude. Rather, it is a dynamic state that, in most people, can be changed for the better, no matter how many years they've lived or how they may have neglected their body in the past.

50 Plus named tournament bicyclist Fred Knoller a top athlete in 1981, at age 86.

Nature gives us a second chance to correct the sins we have committed against our bodies. Your body can be rejuvenated at any time in your life. Whether you are middle-aged or pushing 80, you can regain the vigor, vitality, muscular strength, and aerobic endurance you thought were gone forever.

Dr. Walter M. Bortz II studied the effects of bed rest and concluded that at least a portion of the changes commonly attributed to aging are, in reality, caused by immobility. As such, they're subject to correction by mobility—meaning activity and exercise. In his article published in the *Journal of the American Medical Association,* he stated: "Through the long eons in which our forebears were physically active as a necessity of survival, they died of starvation, injury, and infection. In our current golf-cart age, in which two of these major historic killers are largely controlled, we die of degenerative diseases, on which the impact of our physical inactivity may be considerable.

"'Use it or lose it' is a pervasive biologic law, the application of which has received insufficient attention where the human body is concerned. Medicine particularly has been slow to recognize the benefits of exercise in a number of disease states."[1]

Bortz's personal experience with bed rest and disuse occurred following an Achilles tendon tear he suffered which resulted in his right leg being placed in a cast for six weeks. Although only 35 at that time, he noted his leg resembled that of a man in his seventies. The pain, withering, and stiffness he observed prompted his interest in this field of investigation.

Exercise is enjoyable, easily incorporated into your lifestyle, cost-free, and guaranteed to positively affect your health and longevity. Your single biggest physical defense against aging is exercise. If you did nothing else different, but incorporated some type of regular exercise into your schedule, you would ensure a life unencumbered by reduced energy and illness.

The U.S. Department of Agriculture's Human Nutrition Center on Aging (HNRCA) at Tufts University feels that no group in our population can benefit more from exercise than senior citizens. The muscles of elderly people are just as responsive to weight lifting as those of younger people. When a group of 60- and 70-year-old men participated in a 12-week program of strength training, the results were not only a substantial increase in strength (their lifting ability went from 44 to 85 pounds), but also in muscles that were larger and leaner, with less fat in and around them. An 8-week study of 87- to 96-year old women confined to a nursing home showed that resistance exercises tripled their muscles' strength and increased their size by 10 percent.

Other studies conducted by HNRCA showed that younger-old subjects (those following regular exercise programs) increased their strength by almost 200 percent and their muscle mass by some 15 percent; and the old-old group—the frail elderly—increased strength by as much as

1 Walter M. Bortz II, "Disuse and Aging," *Journal of the American Medical Association* 248, No. 10 (September 10, 1982): 1203–8.

180 percent and muscle mass by up to 12 percent. In terms of overall physical function, elderly study participants regularly experience increases as large as 50 percent. A significant percent of the loss of muscle as we age is preventable, and even reversible!

Research at Baltimore's Gerontology Research Center offers direct evidence, for instance, that "the tendency of the aging heart to stiffen, to take longer to contract, and to spend less time relaxed can be overcome by a relatively light exercise regimen."[2] Prolonged exercise lowers total cholesterol levels and elevates high-density lipoproteins, the form of cholesterol that protects against the buildup of fatty deposits. The bottom line is exercise can protect us from disease.

Seventy-eight-year-old Leslie Pawson (a three-time winner of the Boston Marathon in the 1930s) was the person selected to light the torch signaling the beginning of the Senior Olympics held at Brown University in Providence, Rhode Island, in 1982. Competing with other men in the 65-and-over category, he was the first-place winner in the 6.2-mile run. Clocking 51.54 minutes, he beat out two competitors who were more than a decade younger.

Pawson is an outstanding example of the older person as athlete, but he and many more hundreds of thousands of older people also exemplify by their lives a most important point: that an active life is the right kind of life for all of us, not just for the young. Leslie Pawson is a perfect example of the phrase, "use it or lose it."

Logic dictates that if exercise is beneficial and rejuvenates the body, then inactivity should accelerate the aging process. Studies show just that. The biochemical profile of healthy individuals confined to bed rest due to physical injuries begins to resemble that of people much older. Subjects have been reported who aged as much as ten years physiologically when confined to 36 weeks of bed rest!

Inactivity has been demonstrated to take a considerable toll on heart function, bones, the blood nerves, body composition, brain waves, and

---

2 National Institute on Aging, "With the Passage of Time: the Baltimore Longitudinal Study of Aging." *NIH* Pub. No. 93 (Washington: U.S. Govt Printing Office, 1993).

the immune system when astronauts, prisoners and hospital patients were studied. To take years off your body's age, to keep yourself alert and your immune system strong, exercise.

Aerobics and Isotonic Exercise

There are two major types of exercises. One type is labeled aerobic exercise, more commonly called "aerobics." This is a fast-paced activity that results in heavy energy expenditure. It places demands on your body's cardiovascular apparatus and, over time, produces beneficial changes in your respiratory and circulatory systems. Examples of aerobic exercise are brisk walking, jogging, cycling, swimming, aerobic dance, cross-country skiing, skipping rope, and many recreational sports.

Isotonic exercise constitutes the second major group. This is a strength-building form of exercise built around flexibility-oriented activities such as weight lifting and slow stretching. It focuses on the joints and muscles. These exercises require contraction of a set of muscles, often while you're moving a joint. Some mild recreational sports such as shuffleboard, archery, and horseshoes fall into this category. When most people think of isotonics, they envision muscular conditioning and bodybuilding.

All you need to do is expend more than 1,000 calories each week beyond your basic needs. If you do this, your body will respond with better health and longevity. If you are not now exercising, you should start gradually. Your goal should be to exercise for an hour or so, three to four times each week.

Many activities will fulfill this requirement. Consider some of the activities listed in the following chart compiled by the National Institute of Health. The chart is calculated for a 150-pound individual; deduct one-third of the calories shown for a 100-pound person or add one-third more calories for a 200-pound individual.

Activity (one hour)	Calories burned
Running 10 mph	1,280
Jogging 7 mph	920
Jumping rope	750
Jogging 5½ mph	740
Cross-country skiing	700
Running in place	650
Skiing, 10 mph	600
Squash and handball	600
Swimming 50 yds/min	500
Walking 4½ mph	440
Bicycling 12 mph	410
Tennis (singles)	400
Wood chopping or sawing	400
Square dancing, volleyball, roller skating	350
Walking 3 mph	320
Bowling	270
Golf, lawn-mowing (power mower)	250
Gardening	220
Domestic work	180
Standing	140
Driving an automobile	120
Sitting	100
Lying down or sleeping	80

Other activities that can help burn up calories and that can be fun are: walking the dog, taking a Saturday hike, playing with children, or doing yoga.

The important thing to remember is that these exercise activities must be done *on a regular basis*. Other factors to be aware of in regard to exercise are:

- University of New Hampshire researchers found that exercising increases the rate at which we burn calories after we stop.

- Exercising lowers our body's set point—the preset level of fat the body attempts to maintain regardless of the number of calories consumed—and aids in losing weight permanently.

- Exercising increases and maintains muscle tissue, and decreases excess body fat.

- Exercising will lower our cholesterol if we lose weight during training.

- Exercising lowers blood pressure and reduces our risk of heart attacks.

- Exercising helps you to live longer and better.

Every hour that you sit or lie around instead of being active shortens your life. Workers in high-activity jobs have less coronary artery disease than their low-activity colleagues. According to the *Journal of American Geriatrics*, if an inactive 70-year-old were to begin an exercise program of "moderate activity," the result would be a gain of 15 years life expectancy. If the subject were to achieve the "athlete" level of conditioning, there would be a potential improvement of 40 years.

To get the most out of exercising and protect your body, I suggest:

- Weigh yourself before exercising and drink enough water following exercising to return your weight to its previous level.

- Decrease your intake of coffee and other caffeinated beverages.

- Never drink alcohol before exercising.

- Drink more fluids if you notice your urine is dark. This is an indication of dehydration.

Warm Up and Cool Down when Exercising

Always warm up prior to exercising and cool down following physical activity to prevent or lessen soreness and stiffness the following day.

Warm-ups, cool-downs, and stretches are vital. A 10-minute walk or slow bike ride to wherever you're exercising, or a few minutes of light jogging in place will serve for a warm-up. The idea is to get your blood pumping, start your heartbeat and breathing toward the rates you're going to ask of them, and switch your muscles from an anaerobic to an aerobic mode.

Stretching muscles after a warm-up will help prevent muscle tears and joint injury. Researchers recommend no less than 15 minutes of stretching before exercise for people older than 35. Well-stretched muscles will suffer less from pulls and strains.

After doing your cooling-off stretches, walk around for a few minutes. Then head for the nearest bathtub, or better yet, a hot tub. Sink into the steaming water and let yourself completely r-e-l-a-x. The heat of the water will open up your blood vessels, and your muscles will begin to stretch out. Do not stay in a spa or hot tub for more than 5 minutes, however; your muscles will tense up and contract.

Many people enjoy the addition of a home whirlpool attachment to their bathtub—which offers gentle massage along with the benefits of heat. Some people also like to take a relaxing bath before exercising—or if not a bath, then a hot shower using a massage shower head. Relaxed muscles are less frequently injured than tense ones, so a hot soak makes perfect sense.

Warming-Up/Cooling-Down Exercises

- Lie on the floor on your back, with both knees bent. Close your eyes, take a deep breath, and slowly exhale. Slide one knee forward till your leg is flat. Breathe deeply. Then bend it again. Repeat movement with other leg. Tighten both fists, then let go. Next, take a deep breath. Exhale slowly. Then shrug as you inhale and relax your shoulders as you exhale. Roll your head slowly from side to side.

- Still lying down with knees flexed, slowly bring your right knee as close to your chest as you can. Then put your foot on the floor and slide your leg flat. Return to flexed position. Now repeat with the other leg.

- Lie on your right side with your head on your arm. Keep both knees flexed and hips loose. Slide your left knee as close to your head as comfortably possible, then slowly extend the leg until it is completely straight. Repeat twice, then turn to your left side and do the exercise with your right leg.

- Kneel, resting on your hands and knees. Arch your back and drop your head at the same time. Then reverse the arch by bringing your head up and forming a U with your spine.

- On all fours, move your hands 12 inches forward. At the same time, move your hips back, thus lowering your head and shoulders. Your pectoral muscles will stretch as your chest moves closer to the floor.

- Lie on your back, both knees flexed. Bring your left knee up to your chest. Extend your leg, pointing the toe. Keep your knee locked. Lower this straight leg to the floor, then slide it back to a bent position. Repeat for the right leg. Do the exercise again, this time pointing the toe toward your head.

- Stand with your feet together. Relax by inhaling and exhaling deeply. Drop your head, shoulders, and back gradually. Let gravity help you. Bend your knees and return to standing position. Repeat 2 or 3 times.

Stretching

Calf Stretch

Sitting on the floor, with your feet about a foot apart, loop a towel around the ball of your foot. Without locking your knee, but holding it straight and steady, pull the ends of the towel toward you by leaning back. When you feel the stretch in your calf muscle, hold it for about 15 seconds. If it hurts, let up, or don't hold it as long. Alternate feet for 2 to 4 stretches. Gradually work up to 30-second stretches.

Wall Lean

Move on to the wall lean for further stretching of the calves after you have mastered the towel stretch. With your feet 2 to 3 inches apart, stand 3 to 5 feet from the wall. Put your hands on the wall directly in front of you and bend your elbows until your forearms are resting against the wall. Your feet should be positioned as far as possible from the wall with your heels on the floor and your legs straight. After holding the position for 1 to 15 seconds, walk toward the wall and relax. The wall lean is fairly tough, so repeat it only 3 or 4 times. Over time you may build up to stretches as long as a minute.

Back Stretch

Sit in an armless chair with your feet about a foot apart. Bend forward, bringing your arms and shoulders between your knees. Lean forward as if you were going to put your elbows on the floor. Repeat the stretch several times and gradually build up your holding time.

Bath Stretch

One relaxing way to stretch tired legs is in a bathtub full of warm water. Sitting in the tub with your legs straight, bend forward slowly until you feel the stretch in the muscles at the back of your legs. Relax, keep breathing normally, and hold the stretch for at least 50 or 60 seconds.

Side Stretch

Sit in a chair with your feet 12 inches apart and bend your body to the right, imagining as you do that you are lifting upward against the bend. Don't hold this stretch, just repeat on the left side, then go back to the right. Bend 5 times on each side. As the stretch becomes easier, add more weight to it by holding your hands behind your head as you bend. For even more weight later on, hold your hands above your head as you bend.

Inner Thigh Stretch

For this stretch, you need an empty wall about 6 feet wide. Lie on your back with your legs stretched against the wall, at a 90-degree angle to your body. Your buttocks and heels should be touching the wall. With your knees slightly bent, open your legs as far as they will go. Let gravity do most of the work of pulling your legs down. Hold that position as long as you feel comfortable, up to 5 minutes at a time.

Neck Stretch

While either sitting or standing, clasp your hands behind your neck and let your head fall forward. Hold that position for 10 to 15 seconds, then raise your head and rest. Repeat the stretch, only this time hold your hands an inch higher at the base of your skull. That is the maximum stretch, and should be done only if it is comfortable.

Yoga Stretches

Asana 1

Lie face down, chin resting on the floor, feet stretched out and together, arms relaxed at the sides. Clasp your hands behind your back, take a deep breath and exhale as you lift the upper torso high off the floor. Keep buttocks tightened as you come up. Tilt your head back and pull down strongly with your clasped hands so that the stretch is felt from your neck down to your shoulders, and right into the small of your back. Hold this position without breathing for a few seconds, then breathe out and slowly lower your torso and head to the starting position. Release your hands from the clasped position, turn your head sideways and rest your cheek on the floor. Repeat 3 times.

Asana 2

From a face-down position, with your forehead resting on the floor, stretch your arms far in front of your head. Take a deep breath and lift your torso, head, and arms high off the floor. Do not allow your head or chin to drop. Keep buttocks tightened. Hold this position briefly and then lower your arms and torso to the floor on an exhaled breath. Relax and repeat this exercise once more.

When you decide to incorporate an exercise regimen, it is important to select a combination of exercises that will hold your interest and provide as much of each benefit as possible. An example of excellent exercises that meet these requirements are swimming, biking, cross-country skiing, and jogging.

To maintain good health and promote longevity, I recommend the equivalent of thirty minutes of brisk walking every other day for aerobic benefits, coupled with stretching and flexibility exercises on off days. The "equivalent" can be anything that causes deep breathing and sweating, without causing great discomfort.

Aerobics

One of the main benefits of doing aerobics is that it helps us build stamina. We become conditioned to engage in more strenuous activity over a greater length of time and with less fatigue by regularly doing these exercises.

In order to qualify as aerobic, an activity must be vigorous and sustained for 15 to 30 minutes. Jogging, swimming, bicycling, brisk walking, and dancing definitely qualify. Bowling, golf, and tennis (unless they result in continuous movement) are not aerobic activities.

To warm up for aerobic dancing, extend your arms. Make big circles, keeping your head centered between them. Reach toward the floor and to the ceiling. Keep your lower body still. Breathe deeply.

Another movement consists of quickly shifting your weight from one leg to the other. The movement is light and bouncy. Arms swing in same direction as weight change.

Jog forward 3 steps, then, with hands on hips, bring one knee up. Jog back 3 steps, then bring the other knee up. Alternate the starting leg and repeat this procedure.

Calisthenics

Calisthenics are designed to build up your muscle strength and endurance. They are not meant to strengthen your heart or give you more lung power (respiratory capacity), so they don't qualify as aerobic. Calisthenic exercises strengthen your muscles, give you staying power and help you to become flexible. In order for them to benefit you, however, you must do them regularly. Go through the sequence slowly; don't use jerky movements because they will defeat your purpose.

Breathe deeply and avoid holding your breath while you are doing calisthenics. Do each of these exercises four times daily. As with all exercise, warm up and cool down at each session.

Stomach and Hip Twist

(Lie down, resting on elbows.)
   1. Bring both feet toward hips.

   2. Raise your knees toward your chest and twist them to the left.

   3. Return your feet to the floor and straighten your legs.

   4. Repeat and twist to the right.

   5. Repeat Steps 1–4 from 2–10 times.

For the Hips

(Get down on all fours.)

1. Raise your right knee to the side (hip height) 4–20 times.

2. Lower your knee to the floor.

3. Raise your left knee to the side (hip height) 4–20 times.

4. Lower it to the floor.

5. As the exercise becomes easier, extend your leg out and then return before lowering it.

For the Stomach and Buttocks

(Still on all fours.)

1. Raise your right knee to your chest.

2. Swing your right leg back and lift.

3. Repeat 4–20 times.

4. Repeat Steps 1–3 with the left leg.

For the Total Hip

(Lie down, resting on elbows.)

1. While keeping the left leg as straight as possible, raise and lower it 4–20 times.

2. Roll to the right side and continue to raise and lower the left leg 4–20 times.

3. Roll over on your stomach and continue to raise and lower the left leg 4–20 times.

4. Repeat in reverse for the right leg, 4–20 times.

Stomach and Hip Flexers

(Lie down, resting on elbows.)

1. Bring both feet toward hips.

2. Raise your knees toward your chest while bringing your feet off the floor.

3. Return your feet to the floor and straighten your legs.

4. Repeat 4–20 times. As the exercise becomes easier, try to keep your feet off the floor for the entire set.

For the Stomach

(Lie on your back with knees bent and your feet securely tucked under a chair. Extend your arms over your head, next to your ears.)

1. Swing your arms up and toward your knees while raising your head and shoulders off the floor.

2. Touch your hands to your knees (right-right, left-left).

3. Lower your head and shoulders to the floor as you return your arms to the starting position.

4. Repeat Steps 1–3 and twist to the left.

5. Repeat Steps 1–3 and twist to the right.

6. Repeat Steps 1–5 from 2–10 times.

For the Middle and Upper Back

(Lie on your stomach with a pillow under your hips, hands behind your head and your feet under a chair.)

1. Slowly raise your head, shoulders, and chest as high as possible and then lower them immediately. (Slow, even motion.)

2. Repeat Step 1 and twist to the left.

3. Repeat Step 1 and twist to the right.

4. Repeat Steps 1–3 from 2–10 times.

Walking

Walking provides many of the benefits of more strenuous activities, without much exertion. For this activity, you can progress at your own pace, no equipment is required and you can walk alone or with friends.

The benefits of walking are:

- It promotes more restful sleep.

- A reduction of tension and stress.

- Weight reduction. You burn up 320 calories per hour by walking 3 miles per hour. For every 11 hours of walking you will lose one pound (3500 calories equals one pound).

- Walking improves circulation and is good cardiovascular exercise.

- Improves the ability to take in oxygen.

Tips for Walking

- Walk with your head erect and your stomach in.

- Walk on your whole foot.

- Avoid walking when it is very hot or cold.

- Let your arms swing freely.

- Begin with a 15- to 20-minute walk and walk at a slower pace for the first several minutes as a warm-up.

- Use the best running shoes you can afford. Buy these in a store that specializes in running equipment. Select shoes that are about one-quarter inch longer than your longest toe. The sole must be flexible and the heel counter (the part that wraps around the back of your heel) should be firm.

Other Daily Exercises

- Preparing Dinner—A woman burns up about 105 calories and a man 135 per hour.

- Painting a Wall—You can burn from 165 to 210 calories per hour.

- Washing Windows—Housework such as this burns between 195 and 250 calories per hour.

- Hand Carpentry—Hand sawing burns 305 to 390 calories per hour.

- Doing the Laundry—In addition to having clean clothes, you will burn 190 to 245 calories an hour.

- Gardening—Digging, hoeing, spading, and weeding uses 350 calories an hour for the average woman and 390 calories an hour for the average man.

- Mowing the Lawn—You burn 145 calories an hour steering a ride-on mower and 250 calories per hour pushing a regular lawn-mower.

Water Exercise

These exercises are fun and enhance muscle strength and tone, as well as overall stamina. They're particularly effective in promoting flexibility, coordination and circulation.

Scissors Split

- Float on your stomach, holding on to the side of the pool, with your legs apart.

- Bring your legs together like a pair of scissors, making them overlap before spreading them again. Keep your legs straight.

Repeat 10 times; work up to 25. The splits are good for your thighs, hips, and lower back.

Ballet Stretch

- Stand at a right angle to the pool side, holding on to the edge, with both arms extended.

- Bring your leg up to meet your hand.

- Bring your arm over your head to the side of the pool.

- Bring your leg down. Repeat 10 times, then switch sides. This exercise can be enhanced by using floats around your ankles to give your lower anatomy a more demanding workout.

Twister

- With your back to the pool wall, reach back and hold the rim. Let your legs stretch out in front of you.

- Keeping your legs together, rotate them from side to side like a reversible drill with the hiccups. Repeat 10 times; work up to 40. This firms your waist, hips, and thighs.

Praying Mantis

- Stand in the middle of the pool where your swinging arms won't slug anyone. Keep your arms straight out to the sides.

- Bring your arms down into the water until your hands touch your thighs.

- Bring your hands out in front of you, lifting your arms to the surface. Repeat 10 times; work up to 25. For best results, keep your arms straight, and wear floats around your wrists. This strengthens your arms and upper back muscles.

Weight Lifting

The best exercises are those you enjoy doing, that can be done in moderation throughout life, and that benefit the heart and lungs as well as muscles. Weight lifting doesn't meet these criteria, but it does build strength, tones and shapes muscles, and, in moderation, can be an important part of an overall exercise program.

The following are recommendations from sports experts for incorporating weight lifting into your exercise regimen:

- Focus on building your muscle bulk for the first two months. Have as your goal the ability to do 12–20 repetitions of a lift without undue strain.

- Work on endurance for the next two months. You should be able to do 40–50 repetitions without stopping.

- Lastly, build your strength. Move on to heavier weights that challenge you to do 2–6 repetitions. Increase the amount of the weights as your strength increases.

LIFESTYLE CHANGES TO PRESERVE YOUTH

Many people seek a miraculous "wonder drug" or the Fountain of Youth that so evaded Ponce de Leon, but keep in mind that no substance, technique, or treatment has been accepted and validated as a guaranteed anti-aging remedy, backed up by the kind of thoroughgoing research demanded by the scientific community. This chapter will present some recommendations that are based on both scientific and clinical studies, and logical extensions of that evidence, to assist you in your youthing program.

Armand Hammer was still running his multibillion-dollar empire in his 90s.

The principles and specific references to lifestyle changes given here are based on the subjective testimony of those who have tried them, including my personal successful application of these recommendations.

As an ethical, alternative medical practitioner I encourage you to seek the advice of your own physician on the material I present. Be prepared for him or her to reject and/or ridicule what is given here. Unless your doctor has kept up with alternative medicine literature, he or she will likely "play it safe" and advise you to continue with "business as usual."

There is nothing harmful about anything I discuss, except not incorporating these techniques into your life. For example, many of you are beginning to notice the early signs of aging and are justifiably concerned. Consider the following:

- Between 25 and 35, do you notice you sleep later on weekends than you once did? Is it harder to get up for work on a weekday? As your metabolism slows, do you find it difficult to keep your weight down? Do you notice it is more difficult to play sports or stay out late without paying a price for it the following day?

- Between 35 and 45 you may have been exposed to a friend or family member severely ill, disabled, or who has died. This may refocus your reading toward health issues. Your doctor may be concerned about a "potential problem." If you are a parent, you may be thinking you have only a finite amount of time left in your own life.

- Between 55 and 65 you probably accept a certain amount of aging signs as normal. You learn to live with the aches and pains of arthritis, heart disease, back problems, and so on. Do you get depressed as you ponder your own pending death?

Drugs

Alcohol is a drug, make no mistake about it. Current evidence suggests that moderate drinking won't hurt us, unless we are allergic to alcohol or have a tendency to alcoholism. In fact, it appears even to be good for us; statistics suggest that light drinking decreases our long-range risk of heart attacks. All reports demonstrate that chronic heavy drinking can result in chronic gastrointestinal malfunction as well as extensive organ damage to the liver, pancreas, heart, and brain.

Illegal drugs such as marijuana, cocaine, heroin, and others are all considered bad for us, though heroin is regarded as the most toxic and addictive, as well as the most menacing to other members of society, while of those mentioned marijuana is the least harmful. Using these drugs will cause you to age faster. Just thinking about the possibility of getting "busted" by the authorities for possession of these illegal substances is enough to add a few gray hairs to your head.

Great Sex at Any Age

According to Robert N. Butler, M.D., and Myrna I. Lewis, in *Sex After Sixty,* "women in good health who were able to have orgasms in their younger years can continue to have orgasms until very late in life, well into the eighties."[1] Other studies show that levels of the male sex hormone testosterone do not decrease with age—those with the highest testosterone levels were also those who maintained the highest levels of sexual activity.

If you want to maximize your sex life, I suggest the following:

- Cut down on your alcohol intake. The more alcohol consumed, the more problematic sex becomes. Alcohol lowers the testosterone level in men, creating potency problems; in women it delays orgasm.

- Add more zinc to your diet. Zinc is helpful in the maintenance of male sexual health and vigor, according to Georgetown University researchers. Smoking and drinking depletes our ability to use zinc. Liver, sunflower seeds, oats, nuts, and cheese are good sources of zinc.

- Exercise regularly. The more active you are, the greater will be your vigor and interest in sex, both mentally and physically.

- Cut down on sweets. Hypoglycemia (low blood sugar) has been connected with potency problems in men and orgasm difficulties in women.

- Question your physician about prescription medication you may be taking. Some drugs can lead to impotence (in men) or a lessening of sexual desire (in both sexes). Tranquilizers and antidepressants sometimes fall into this category, as do some drugs used to control high blood pressure. The dosages of necessary medication can sometimes be reduced to lessen these side effects.

---

1   Robert N. Butler, *Sex After Sixty: A Guide for Men and Women for Their Later Years* (Boston: Hall, 1976).

- Cut down on coffee; caffeine affects the entire nervous system, including sexual functioning. Consider switching to herb tea.

Sunlight

I have briefly discussed the aging effects of exposure to the sun before. In this section we will discuss how to protect ourselves from this aging accelerator in greater detail.

Sunlight ages us by reacting with oxygen in our cells, forming free radicals (see chapter 6). These unstable oxygen molecules damage many components of our cells, such as their membranes, fats, the proteins the cells need to operate, and the DNA and RNA they need to replicate. This can result in the following changes to our skin:

- Spotting with brown patches, red spidery veins, and warty growths.

- Accelerating by many times the normal loss of elasticity.

- Changing the skin's color from rosy red to yellowish.

- Toughening, roughening, and wrinkling extensively.

Too much sun, according to a study at Cornell Medical School, can deplete your body's stores of the very beta-carotene that protects it. The best advice I can give you is to stay out of the sun as much as possible.

If you live in a warm climate as I do, with the Los Angeles sun shining just about every day and at high temperatures, you may out of necessity or desire be out in the sun. Always use sunscreen lotions to protect your skin.

Sunscreens are excellent at absorbing or blocking the ultraviolet B (UV) light rays that can cause a sunburn. The sun protection factor (SPF) is the most important consideration when choosing a sunscreen.

Ultraviolet A (UVA) light has recently been linked to the sun's aging effect. Where the UVB rays penetrate only the top layers of the skin, the more powerful UVA rays penetrate even deeper, damaging the deepest layers of the skin and the supporting collagen tissues. I suggest you use a sunscreen that contains both para-aminobenzoic acid (PABA) and oxybenzone. When reading the sunscreen label understand that the sun protection factor listed on the bottle or tube applies only to its UVB (sunburn) protection. When it comes to the damaging UVA rays, their protection value is equivalent to about a 2. The usual range is 2 to 15 for the UVB. Always go for the highest UVB rating.

If you are concerned that you might be allergic to PABA, be assured that laboratory tests show that fewer than one person in a thousand has documented allergic reactions to PABA. You can purchase sunscreens without PABA if you are the rare person with such an allergy. For example, you can obtain Sundown Broad Spectrum, because it uses titanium, which blocks UVA rays, and is free of PABA.

To summarize, if you must be in the sun, use wide-spectrum sunscreens containing PABA and oxybenzone. If the PABA bothers your skin, switch to another sunscreen with an equal SPF number, and preferably one that contains oxybenzone for UVA protection.

Smoking

This section could be completed in two words, don't smoke. One fact that the public sometimes misses is that the major cause of decreased life expectancy as a result of smoking cigarettes is not cancer; it is heart disease.

Here are some interesting longevity conclusions made from recent studies regarding smoking:

- Smokers die faster than nonsmokers, at every age and with the increased number of cigarettes smoked, and smokers die at a greater rate from every disease.

- Nonsmoking wives or husbands of cigarette smokers have a lowered life expectancy.

- One-pack-a-day smokers have twice the chance of nonsmokers of dying from age fifty to sixty. Two-pack-a-day smokers have three times the chance.

- On the average, smokers die about eight years younger than non-smokers.

Pets

One of the best ways to live longer and healthier, while being the recipient of unconditional love, is to own a pet. Pets enhance our physical and emotional health. A University of Maryland Hospital study revealed that after one year, only three of 53 patients who were pet owners had died. Of the 39 other patients who didn't have any pets, 11 had died. The key to these results wasn't simply that the dog owners received more exercise and were therefore healthier. When dog owners were eliminated from the study, 10 other pet owners who survived after a year were left; the pets were cats, horses, chickens, goldfish, and even one iguana. None of these pet owners exercised their pets, so the key to their survival had to be the owning of the pets rather than any exercise connected with them.

Talking to animals has been shown to lower blood pressure in a study conducted by Aaron Katcher, a psychiatrist at the University of Pennsylvania. Despite the vigor they expended while greeting the animals, the volunteers in Katcher's study nevertheless had significantly lower blood pressure readings while greeting their pets than while reading.[2]

Attentiveness seems to be a key factor in these results. One of the things dog owners prize most about their pets is attentiveness. The dogs make contact—they acknowledge their masters' presence. One could say that the dogs make their masters feel more human—which is hardly stretching the point, since another study has shown that many dog

---

2 A. Katcher and A. Beck, *New Perspectives on Our Lives with Companion Animals* (Philadelphia: University of Pennsylvania Press, 1983).

owners actually see their pets as "human" members of the family rather than merely as companion animals.

Among significant benefits in caring for a pet is maintaining a more regular eating pattern. Older men and women who live alone tend to skip meals, but if they're feeding a pet are more likely to prepare food for themselves too.

Another advantage is exercise. People who live alone sometimes tend to have a hard time getting up in the morning. They become lifeless, lying or sitting around. Owning a pet—particularly a dog that needs to be walked—gives some structure to the day; it forces them to get some fresh air and exercise.

Companionship must not be left out of this list of benefits of pet ownership. Two senior citizens walking their dogs in a park, for instance, are much more apt to stop, chat, and maybe strike up a friendship than if they were taking their strolls alone.

If owning a pet that requires this kind of care and attention is not an option, there are other alternatives. Fish, lava lamps, open fires, and other focusing devices have been shown to reduce high blood pressure. Dr. Katcher says, "Anything that turns your attention outward to the natural environment around you is a powerful way of controlling tension."[3] When you lower your blood pressure you are extending both the quantity and quality of your life.

Keep Your Brain Young

I have previously discussed studies showing that our cognitive functions do not degenerate when we age, unless we engage in self-destructive behavior. A National Institute on Aging study suggested that not remembering things as we age may be less a matter of forgetfulness than of failing to concentrate on what we're doing. The study further suggested that not paying close attention is usually the cause of forgetfulness when the tasks involved are simple ones.

---

3   Ibid.

Robert L. Kahn, Ph.D., of the University of Chicago, found that many older people complain of having a poor memory, but that their complaints don't jibe with their actual performance on memory tests.[4] We may have a better memory than we think, but downgrade our abilities because we're so worried about losing the memory that we overreact to any little slip.

Emotional depression, bereavement, illness, loneliness, economic worries—all can contribute to a chronic case of the blues and wipe out the memory. A dull life easily can lead to depression and to mental deterioration.

To enhance your memory, also eat the right "brain food." Deficiencies of certain B vitamins can cause disturbances in brain function. For example, a mild thiamine deficiency can bring about memory disturbances, inability to concentrate, insomnia, and a lack of initiative. Beef kidney, brewer's yeast, sunflower seeds, dried soybeans, kidney and other beans all contain thiamine.

Hobbies are one simple way to increase your longevity; there are many options from stamp collecting to raising sheep. Take the case of Alma M. Campbell, who has been raising sheep as a part-time hobby on her Bucks County, Pennsylvania, farm for a good part of her life. "My mother bought me my spinning wheel in 1922 at an auction for 50 cents. She thought I was crazy for wanting it," says Alma, a retired science teacher. "I knew I would use it some day. I had it in back of my head that I just might want to spin the wool from my sheep. When I retired in 1964 I found the time. Raising sheep is a good hobby for a person—a person with a lot of energy," she emphasizes. "The raising is fun, the shearing is work, and the spinning is sheer pleasure."[5]

---

4   R. L. Kahn, *Work and Health* (New York: Wiley, 1981).
5   Ashley Montagu, *Growing Young* (New York: McGraw-Hill, 1981).

Here is a list of some lifestyle changes you can make to facilitate your longevity.

- Make sure you get exercise every few days.
- Learn to eat nutritionally balanced and wholesome meals.
- Take time each week to do something special just for yourself.
- Create a place to relax or be by yourself at home or nearby.
- Learn and use time management techniques in your daily life.
- Stop smoking.
- Learn to use relaxation exercises instead of alcohol or drugs to unwind before sleep.
- Don't bring work home at night.
- Take up a hobby you enjoy.
- Join a group that lets you get out with friends regularly. Work to bring yourself within five pounds of your "ideal" weight.
- Do some form of deep relaxation (hypnosis, meditation, yoga, biofeedback, etc.).

HYPNOTIZE YOURSELF TO A LONGER AND HAPPIER LIFE

I n all the time that I have used hypnosis (since 1974), I have never seen or even heard of a negative effect or situation experienced by a patient. In my experience, the worst that can happen is nothing, i.e., no trance is induced.

Hypnosis is simply a way of relaxing and setting aside the conscious mind while at the same time activating the subconscious mind. Then suggestions can be made directly to the subconscious, enabling the patient to act on these suggestions with greater ease and efficiency.

Hypnosis can be described by the following formula:

Misdirected attention + belief + expectation = hypnosis

The Delaney sisters, Sarah and Elizabeth, at 101 and 103, wrote Having Our Say, the Delaney Sisters First 100 Years.

The Hypnotic Trance

Hypnosis takes place in the alpha state, or subconscious mind, which can be compared to a computer. Just as a computer is programmed or fed information, the subconscious mind is constantly undergoing a programming process. Everything that we can detect through our five senses is permanently stored in the subconscious mind's memory bank.

The term "hypnosis" stems from the Greek word *hypnos,* which literally means sleep.

A subject in a hypnotic trance may appear to be sleeping, but that is where the resemblance ends. Anyone in trance can think, talk, open their eyes, respond to suggestion, and move in any way. In fact, people in hypnosis (notice I did not say under) are usually aware of their surroundings and can hear other sounds besides the voice of the hypnotist.

C. S. Moss, in *Hypnosis in Perspective,* presented a description of what he thought was the "conventional image of hypnosis."

"The subject is asked to seat himself and fixate his gaze on a specific point, often a shiny object, while the operator monotonously intones soothing suggestion[s] of relaxation and drowsiness. If all goes well, in a few minutes the subject's eyelids will droop or flutter and finally close, and he will slump in his chair, apparently deep in sleep....It will be noted that the cooperative subject loses his facial motility, he becomes literal or humorless, and his behavior is characterized by lethargy or psychomotor retardation, as if he were extremely reluctant to think or to move.

"...If told to open his eyes, the subject will often have an unseeing stare....In this condition suggestions may be given for positive or negative hallucinations ('When you open your eyes you will see a little black dog sitting in the corner' or 'Now everyone else has left the room and you and I are alone').

"At the termination of the demonstration, the subject may be instructed to 'forget' all of these events when he awakens. It can also be suggested that later, in response to a prearranged signal from the operator, the subject will engage in some manner of post-hypnotic behavior, such as experiencing an overwhelming thirst when the operator strikes a match. The usual procedure is then to slowly awaken the subject with accompanying suggestions of well-being and comfort."[1]

Hypnosis has been explained in terms of trance states, role playing, conditioning, and ego regression, but no theory is currently widely accepted. I find that much hypnotic behavior can be understood in

---

1   C. S. Moss, *Hypnosis in Perspective* (New York: MacMillan, 1965), pp. 3–4.

terms of biological survival mechanisms. The slowing down and the immobilization of physical and sensory processes is a natural defense mechanism when flight or fight is not possible and this slowing-down process further assists in recovery after trauma.

Hypnosis is not a sharply delineated state, but a fluctuating day-dream process that, like any altered state of awareness, depends on the degree of arousal or perceptivity induced by the hypnotist or the sub-ject. The capacity to enter into hypnosis is as subjective and naturalistic a phenomenon as sleep. Hypnosis cannot be explained by any single factor such as cortical inhibition, hypersuggestibility, dissociation, dependency, or transference because, like any mental process, it is a mixture of several processes occurring at the same time.

Definitions and theories of hypnosis are almost as numerous as the physicians, dentists, psychologists, and lay people who have been inter-ested in it. Most authorities now seem to agree that hypnosis brings about some sort of altered awareness and behavior, as compared with the presumably normal awake state.

A hypnotic state also occurs spontaneously when a person is driving long distances along a straight road that does not require alert behavior. It occurs when we watch rain falling, reading, watching television or a movie and losing track of time, viewing repetitive flashes of light and shadow, and so on. A hypnotic state may also occur spontaneously when people are frightened, disoriented in space, very ill, starving, or experiencing a religious reverie state.

Since hypnosis is 100 percent natural, it is sometimes referred to as a waking dream (daydream) or a working dream (when used to elimi-nate habits or phobias, or to slow down the aging process). Through this natural state we can make use of the unlimited potential of the human mind. Hypnosis is a tool that allows us to use more of our mind and to use it more dynamically and effectively. When we enter into a state of hypnosis, we experience a level of relaxed receptivity with increased perception—a state of deep relaxation which quiets the body and opens the mind. With its defenses down, the mind is especially open to suggestion, the type of which is determined by a person's goals and ideals—the reasons for wanting to use hypnosis.

Alpha is the brain wave characteristic of the hypnotic trance. Our brain automatically enters this alpha state just prior to falling asleep and as we awaken in the morning; many people describe alpha as half-awake and half-asleep.

There are three other brain waves, as measured by the electroencephalograph (EEG). Beta is our normal everyday waking state, theta is exhibited in deep hypnosis, intense meditation, and during the early stages of nighttime sleep, and delta is found in the deepest state of sleep or unconsciousness.

Principles of Hypnosis

When I discuss hypnosis, I refer to *self-hypnosis*. All hypnosis is actually self-hypnosis. It is impossible to hypnotize someone against his or her will, unless certain drugs are used, which I never recommend or use. Thus, during a hypnotic session, a patient learns how to hypnotize him or herself, utilizing the services of a hypnotherapist. The term for this is *heterohypnosis*, meaning hypnosis by another (*hetero* means "other").

The best hypnotic subjects are people who can focus their concentration, are intelligent, can express emotions, are open-minded, have excellent memory, visualize easily, and for whom time passes quickly. The very best hypnotic patients are children between the ages of eight and sixteen. I will work with children as young as five.

Those people who usually make the worst hypnotic patients are people who have very short attention spans, tend to focus on the past and future rather than the present, are overly critical, use logic instead of emotions, have lower I.Q.s and have great difficulty "letting themselves go." Mental retardation, senility, brain damage, inability to understand the language of the hypnotist, and overly cynical attitudes are also going to inhibit the induction of a hypnotic trance.

Our purpose in this chapter is to learn how to use self-hypnosis to slow down the aging process. There are several reasons that hypnosis is employed by therapists such as myself. Weight reduction, the elimination of smoking, improving the immune system and health in general, developing a sense of humor, attracting abundance, instilling a motivation, and preparing for personal changes are but a few of the uses of this dynamic and empowering technique. A more comprehensive list of the goals attainable through hypnosis are:

- Increased relaxation and the elimination of tension.

- Increased and focused concentration.

- Improved memory.

- Improved reflexes.

- Increased self-confidence and assertiveness.

- Pain control.

- Improved sex life.

- Increased organization and efficiency.

- Increased motivation.

- Improved interpersonal relationships.

- Improved ability to set and attain goals.

- Facilitating a better career path.

- Elimination of anxiety and depression.

- Overcoming bereavement.

- Elimination of all types of headaches, including migraine.

- Elimination of allergies and skin disorders.

- Strengthening one's immune system to resist any disease.

- Elimination of habits, phobias, and other "self-defeating sequences."

- Improving decisiveness.

- Overcoming insomnia.

- Improving the quality of people and circumstances in general that you attract in your life.

- Increasing your ability to earn and hold onto money.

- Overcoming obsessive-compulsive behavior.

- Improving the overall quality of your life.

- Improved psychic awareness.

- Establishing and maintaining harmony of body, mind, and spirit.

- Slowing down the aging process.

Here are some additional principles of self-hypnosis you should know:

- Hypnotic programming works by repeated exposure.

- Absolutely everyone can be hypnotized.

- You will remember everything that you experience during a trance, unless you are a very deep level subject.

- The more determined you are to attain a goal, the greater your chances of success.

- You cannot be forced to do anything as a result of hypnosis that you would not normally do.

- You must also have motivation to overcome the difficulty you complain about. It is possible to increase motivation by suggestion.

- If a post-hypnotic suggestion is used (most therapeutic suggestions are post-hypnotic), always incorporate a cue for the termination of the suggestion if it should be ended.

- If the post-hypnotic suggestion should not be terminated, be very careful not to inadvertently give a cue for termination.

- A permissive suggestion is more likely to be carried out than a dominating command.

- Work on only one issue at a time when using autohypnosis.

Suggestion

The key to using hypnosis is to give yourself a verbal or mental instruction to attain a specific goal. We refer to this as a suggestion. If the suggestion is designed to be enacted following the hypnotic trance, the term *posthypnotic suggestion* is applied. Posthypnotic suggestions can be effective at any depth, although the deeper the trance the more likely they are to be carried out.

If your head spontaneously rolls sideways or forward, the hypnotic depth is increasing. Shallow, diaphragmatic breathing usually is associated with lighter stages, while slow, deep, regular abdominal breathing generally is characteristic of deeper stages of hypnosis. Other signs indicative of increasing depth are the blinking and the involuntary drooping of the eyelids. The trembling of the eyelids after closure usually indicates further deepening.

The success of all suggestion depends on gaining cooperation of the subconscious mind, and if it is approached with sincerity and patience, you will be rewarded with a relaxing and empowering state of mind. Some people find that if they spend a minute or two in deep breathing before the relaxation session it helps them to unwind and to "let go" more rapidly.

The following exercise will get you oriented to this relaxed state we call hypnosis:

Make yourself comfortable on a couch or a bed with or without a pillow, as suits you best. Some people find that they can relax better on the floor with a carpet or a rug to lie on, but after experimenting you will be the best judge of what suits your needs. A small flat cushion or pad may also be helpful, either in the small of the back or behind the knees. Spend a little time experimenting until the best conditions conductive to relaxation have been arranged.

When you are satisfied from your experiments that you have found the best conditions in which to be as comfortable as possible, lie on your back with your hands open and arms by your sides, but do not let them touch your body. Just let them lie comfortably at your sides and rest quietly and easily, looking at the ceiling. Don't stare, but concentrate your gaze on one spot. Don't try to do anything else. Close your eyes if it is an effort to keep them open, but do not try to "put yourself under." The object of this resting is to let your mind and body gradually slow down. If your mind starts off on some task of its own, such as making out a shopping list, or working on some problem, bring it back and remind yourself of what you are doing. After a brief interval, particularly if you have been busy previously, you will feel various degrees of tirednesses which you were not conscious of before. You will be able to feel these sensations of tiredness located specifically in various muscles in the arms, legs, hands, back, shoulders, and feet.

The next step is to mentally "feel" each of these in turn. Let yourself relax as far as you can. Then direct your attention to your right hand and let it remain there for about ten seconds, then transfer your attention to your left hand, and then to your right foot, and then to your left foot, again spending about ten seconds on each. After this, transfer your awareness to the sensations present in the muscles of the face, lips, tongue, and mouth. As far as possible, avoid moving any of these parts.

You will find that when you direct your attention to one part of your body, you will forget all the other parts of your body. Go over your hands, feet, and the muscles in your face, as just directed, three times. You will notice as the exercise proceeds that any tensions that may have been present when you commenced the exercise will begin to ease and die down.

Making Your Own Tapes

Before I present several scripts on self-hypnosis, some instruction on making your own personal self-hypnosis tape is in order. Researchers have demonstrated that if appropriate preparations are taken, tape-recorded induction procedures may be almost as effective as the "live" voice of an experienced hypnotist.

Self-hypnosis tapes are tools to build your mind and remodel your life the way you want it to be. They are an idea whose time has come. They will help you develop mental strength and put the "self" back into self-help. In addition, these tapes will accelerate your ability to access your subconscious and slow down the aging process.

Naturally, the room you use for self-hypnosis should be as quiet as possible. I would close the door and inform other people present not to disturb you for at least thirty minutes. I highly recommend headphones when you use pre-recorded tapes. This functions to block out extraneous noise and directs the voice of the hypnotist to the subject's subconscious mind. Other recommendations for your hypnosis room are:

- Keep a blanket by your recliner.

- Keep the temperature of the room slightly above room temperature.

- If you are using an eye fixation device, place it above eye level when you are reclined in your chair.

- A metronome, or a tape of metronome beats, makes an excellent background for inducing hypnosis. It also helps you pace your voice.

At first it seems that the concept of making your own self-hypnosis tape requires skills and time that you may not possess. It also suggests an expensive procedure that may be beyond your budget. In actuality, none of the above assumptions are justified.

You are probably familiar with commercially pre-recorded self-hypnosis tapes. These are inexpensive and allow you to practice this technique in the comfort and privacy of your own home. It is far more desirable for you to make your own tapes because you can personalize a tape for your own specific goals. It is the equivalent of purchasing a custom-designed suit versus one off the rack.

It requires only an hour of your time, on the average, to produce a high-quality self-hypnosis tape. You will also learn more about the art and science of hypnosis by making your own tapes.

There are only three simple steps to creating your own self-hypnosis tape. The first step is the induction into hypnosis. This can be a standard one from the examples that I present in this chapter. Scripts for specific goals constitute the second step, and you will find these throughout this section. Wake up suggestions make up the third and final step and a standardized example is given.

When recording your personalized tape, speak slowly and distinctly. You may find it desirable to play soothing background music while you are recording your tape. The background music can be used to mask over unwanted noise of traffic or voices in another room. Sounds—like ocean waves, gentle rain, or sounds of spring in the country—are available on tapes and records. Other options include using a metronome or the ticking of a clock to pace your voice and facilitate the induction into hypnosis.

By playing your self-hypnosis tapes you will literally be using your subconscious mind to build your future. Self-hypnosis means that you do this building process yourself—there is no middleman, because client and hypnotist are one and the same. With self-hypnosis you are always in complete control because you are the one giving the suggestions and controlling the whole process. You are utilizing more of your mind and applying it in a personal, positive way. Self-hypnosis is a learning and growing experience. It functions as your springboard for constructive change.

You affirm your purpose and goals when you give yourself positive hypnotic suggestions. Practice will soon speed up this process and allow you to become more proficient in self-hypnosis. The addition of visualization exercises (given later in this chapter) allows you to facilitate making these goals a reality. You may look upon this approach as one of reprogramming old obstacles into new opportunities.

The best time to practice self-hypnosis is in the early morning, immediately upon awakening. You may be a night person or experience your energy peaks in the afternoon, but regardless of your biological clock, I have found that the earlier you begin your exercises, the more you obtain from them. The last thing you want to do is to give in to the natural, but dysfunctional, tendency to procrastinate. You can also use self-hypnosis at other times of the day when you want to relax and focus your energies.

When using one of my scripts, or making a customized script yourself, record these suggestions immediately after your standard induction. Depending on your pace and the cycle you choose, your completed tape will be approximately one-half hour in length. Use this tape once or twice each day for one month. Do not record a tape longer than thirty minutes.

Achievement can happen at any time. It can happen immediately or you can experience it later on. Subtle changes usually begin to appear in a few days and substantial changes should be experienced within a few weeks. Some people respond quickly to the message of their tape, other people slowly and carefully change and grow, step by step, day by day. Eventually you will build your confidence and write your own scripts.

Here are some additional tips for more effectively using your tapes.

1. When you are preparing to enter a hypnotic trance, do your fingers show signs of curling? Are your hands tight? Are they

clenched? If so, let your fingers uncurl and relax your hands. Are your legs crossed? Uncrossing them allows for better circulation. Are there any parts of your clothing or shoes that feel tight? Loosen them for your own comfort. Allow yourself to slow down a little more.

2. If you want to take a more active part in your tape session, *sit up* in bed or in a chair and lie down only after the session is finished.

3. For use of your tape at bedtime, do not include a wake-up section. Simply suggest that you go right into your natural sleep cycle from the hypnotic state. I have included a script for insomnia.

4. It is quite natural for your conscious mind to wander during self-hypnosis. Do not be concerned that you might be wasting your time when this happens. You may also experience hypno-amnesia (lack of memory), and this signifies a fairly deep level of hypnosis. Your conscious mind's activities and/or state of boredom is irrelevant to your use of self-hypnosis. We only care about the subconscious.

5. I highly recommend adding music at open spaces throughout the tape. This will deepen your trance level and block out distracting environmental noises. The total time, including the music, should not exceed thirty minutes, as I mentioned earlier.

6. After recording your script on tape, add a wake-up procedure as I have instructed. The term *wake-up* is not accurate, since you are never really asleep or unconscious. I only use this term since it is so ingrained in the public's perception of hypnosis. The purpose of the wake-up section is simply to allow your mind to gradually orient itself back to the everyday conscious world.

Simple Exercise Script

The following script can be used to make your first tape. This is a simple exercise and includes an induction and wake-up components. Use an ocean sound alone for about 10 seconds, then metronome beats in the background, in sync to your voice.

> Sit back and listen to the beats of the metronome in the background. Each beat of the metronome will bring you deeper and deeper into relaxation. Listen as I count backward from 20 to 1. Each count backward will make each and every muscle in your body completely relaxed, until I reach the count of 1 in which you will be in a very deep and relaxed level of hypnosis. 20, 19, 18, deeply, deeply relaxed. 17, 16, 15, down, down, down. 14, 13, 12, very, very deep. 11, 10, 9, deep, deep relaxed. 8, 7, 6, so very sleepy. 5, 4, 3, deeply, deeply relaxed. 2, 1, deep, deep sleep. 20 – 20 – 20. You are now in a deep relaxed level of hypnosis. Listen as I count backward, again this time from 7 to 1. As I count backward from 7 to 1, you are going to hear the beats of the metronome in the background decrease in volume, decrease in volume with each count until I reach the count of 1, in which you will hear nothing but my voice. You will be in a very, very deep and relaxed level of hypnosis.
>
> Decrease metronome beats until the count of 1, when they are gone completely. 7, deeper, deeper, deeper, down, down, down. 6, deeper, deeper, deeper, down, down, down. 5, deeper, deeper, deeper, down, down, down. 4, deeper, deeper, deeper, down, down, down. 3, deeper, deeper, deeper, down, down, down. 2, deeper, deeper, deeper, down, down, down. 1, deeply, deeply, relaxed, deeply, deeply asleep. 20 – 20 – 20. You are now in a nice deep relaxed level of hypnosis. The repetition of the number 20 three times in succession by my voice or your voice will quickly and very deeply get you into this nice deep level of hypnosis. This will get you quicker and deeper each and every time you practice self-hypnosis.

You can add whatever instructions you want to from this point on and end the trance as follows:

Now, in a few moments . . . when I count up to 5 . . . you will open your eyes and be wide awake again.

You will feel much better for this deep, refreshing sleep.

You will feel completely relaxed...both mentally and physically...quite calm and composed...without the slightest feeling of drowsiness or tiredness. And next time...you will not only be able to go into this sleep much more quickly and easily...but you will be able to go much more deeply. One...two...three...four...five...wide awake and refreshed.

Here is a classic eye fixation induction technique you can use:

Now get as comfortable as possible. Rest your head. Rest your head on the back of the chair. Fix your eyes directly above your forehead. Keep looking directly at one spot on the ceiling. Notice now that your eyes are getting very, very *heavy,* your *lids* are getting very, very, very *tired.* Your lids are getting *heavier* and *heavier,* and the heavier your lids get now, the better you will relax your lids. The better you relax your eyelids, the better you will follow all subsequent suggestions. Your lids are getting *heavier* and *heavier.* They are getting *very, very tired.* Your lids are getting *very, very heavy.* Your eyelids are blinking. That is a good sign that the lids are getting *heavier* and *heavier.* Your lids are blinking a little more. That is right. If you really wish to go into a deeper state of relaxation, all you have to do is to let your lids close *tightly,* very tightly, at the count of three. You will close your eyes, not because you have to but because you really wish to go deeper and deeper relaxed. One – your eyelids are getting heavier and heavier. Two – getting much heavier. Your lids are blinking still more. Three – now, *close your eyes tight* and let your eyeballs roll up into the back of your head. As your eyeballs roll up into the back of your head, notice how your lids are sticking tighter together. You feel the tightness, do you not? This shows that it's really beginning to work. And your lids continue to stick tighter and tighter together. And as your eyeballs are rolled up toward your forehead for a few moments longer, you will go deeper and deeper relaxed.

Eye-Fixation Technique Without Sleep Suggestions

I will teach you to relax. You will *relax every fiber, every muscle in your body.* When you raise your right hand, let it fall limply into your lap. Let your hand fall as though it is as heavy as lead, jut like a wet dish towel. Your arm is completely relaxed. Breathe in deeply and relax your diaphragm. Again. Now relax your feet and legs the same you did your hands. Make them *very, very heavy.* I want you to feel a very pleasant tingling, relaxed feeling in your toes. It will travel up from the soles of your feet, up your legs to your abdomen and chest." (Pause.) Take another deep breath and relax still more. Again. Now relax your lower jaw . . . more . . . Relax your cheeks. Now your eyes are very tired and heavy. They are closing, closing, closing. Close your eyes.

Relax your forehead. Listen only to my voice. You can think of anything you wish, but you will concentrate on my voice. I want you to go into an even deeper state of relaxation. 1, 2, 3, . . . *deep, deeply relaxed.* . . .every muscle from your head to your toes is completely relaxed. You will remain relaxed until I ask you to open your eyes. When you open your eyes, you will be completely relaxed and full of confidence. Each time you practice self-hypnosis, you will always relax quickly and deeply with this method. You will never forget these suggestions.

When I count to 3, you will open your eyes and be completely relaxed, feeling fine. 1, 2, 3, wide awake and refreshed and eyes open.

Insomnia

It is desirable to rid yourself of insomnia to facilitate incorporating this youthing program. Researchers inform us that two out of every ten women have some form of insomnia, while only one in every ten men experience this.

The REM (rapid eye movement) phase of our five-stage sleep cycle is where all dreaming, hypnosis programming, and "cleansing" (to be described shortly) techniques are applied. You can see why it is so important to eliminate insomnia.

There are three types of sleep disturbances:

- Type I insomnia is characterized by requiring more than 30 minutes to fall asleep. This is also called sleep onset insomnia.

- Type II, or sleep maintenance insomnia, is particularly frustrating since you wake up periodically throughout the night (usually every 1½ to 2 hours—during the REM phase).

- Type III insomnia is the most disturbing and it is characterized by the inability to get back to sleep after you are awakened at four or five in the morning, several hours before you are scheduled to wake up. Researchers call this early-morning awakening insomnia.

The following script will assist you in eliminating insomnia once and for all:

As you become more able to cope with and face up to the situations that have been causing your anxiety, then you will begin to sleep more easily and more soundly. There are no serious consequences to insomnia and the worries about the consequences of not sleeping are one of the main causes of this problem. If you do fall asleep, so much the better! If you don't…it doesn't matter, because sooner or later you will.

Associate this relaxed feeling with bedtime relaxation. As a result of this treatment you will feel more relaxed, less tense and less anxious each day. As bedtime approaches you will feel more and more pleasantly tired. You will go to bed at the same time each night and as soon as you put your head on the pillow you will begin to relax. You will no longer worry whether you are going to sleep or not. You will devote all of your attention to totally relaxing. You are steadily losing your desire to wake up in the middle of the night…you are steadily increasing your desire to fall asleep quickly and sleep through the night undisturbed.

After you are in bed, and just before you drop off to natural sleep, you will place yourself into a self-hypnotic trance by taking a deep breath, holding it to the count of 6, letting it out slowly and repeating the number 20, three times in succession, and then tell yourself that there is no need to take the day's problems to bed with you. As far as you are concerned, bed is for restful and healthful sleep without dreams or thoughts that will disturb either your rest or your health. If you find yourself reliving a problem or negative situation, whether real or imaginary, you will put it out of your mind immediately and relax totally. You will reward yourself with this feeling of relaxation which feels so very good.

Now imagine a scene that you find most pleasant…a scene that you would rather be in if you had a choice…as soon as your head touches the pillow at night you will re-create this positive scene and enter into hypnosis, then quickly into natural sleep. If you should awaken in the middle of the night you will not be disturbed…simply take a deep breath, hold it to the count of six, let it out slowly and repeat the number 20, three times, and you will enter into hypnosis again and then quickly drift into natural sleep.

You will fall asleep promptly and sleep soundly and restfully throughout the night. You will awaken in the morning refreshed, wide awake, well rested and ready to start the day.

Self-Confidence

Building up your self-confidence is an important step in youthing. You want to enlist the aid of the subconscious mind to mobilize every resource in your quest to slow down the aging process. This script will be useful in that regard:

Every day...you will become physically stronger and fitter. You will become more alert...more wide awake...more energetic. You will become much less easily tired...much less easily fatigued...much less easily discouraged.

Every day...your nerves will become stronger and steadier.

You will become so deeply interested in whatever you are doing...so deeply interested in whatever is going on...that your mind will become much less preoccupied with yourself...and you will become much less conscious of yourself...and your own feelings.

Every day...your mind will become calmer and clearer...more composed...more placid...more tranquil. You will become much less easily worried...much less easily agitated...much less fearful and apprehensive...much less easily upset.

You will be able to think more clearly...you will be able to concentrate more easily...your memory will improve...and you will be able to see things in their true perspective...without magnifying them...without allowing them to get out of proportion.

Every day...you will become emotionally much calmer...much more settled...much less easily disturbed. And, every day...you will enjoy a greater feeling of personal well-being...a greater feeling of personal safety and security...than you have felt for a long, long time. Every day...you will become...and you will remain...more and more completely relaxed...both mentally and physically.

And as you become...and as you remain...more relaxed...and less tense each day...so you will develop much more confidence in yourself...much more confidence in your ability to do...not only what you have to do each day...but also much more confidence in your ability to do what you ought to be able to do…without fear of failure…without fear of consequences…without anxiety…without uneasiness. Because of this…every day…you will feel more and more independent…more able to "stick up for yourself"…to stand on your own two feet…to hold your own no matter how difficult or trying things may be.

Every day, in every way, you are getting better, better, and better…Negative thoughts and negative suggestions have no influence over you at any mind level.

And, because all these things will happen…exactly as I tell you they will happen…you are going to feel much happier…much more contented…much more cheerful…much more optimistic…much less easily discouraged…much less easily bothered.

As you become more relaxed and less tense each day…so…you will remain more relaxed and less tense…when you are in the presence of other people…no matter whether they be few or many…no matter whether they be friends or strangers.

You will be able to meet them on equal terms…and you will feel much more at ease in their presence…without the slightest feeling of inferiority…without becoming self-conscious…without becoming embarrassed or confused…without feeling that you are making yourself conspicuous in any way.

You will become so deeply interested…so deeply absorbed in what you are doing and saying…that you will concentrate entirely on this to the complete exclusion of everything else.

Because of this…you will remain perfectly relaxed…perfectly calm and self-confident…and you will become much less conscious of yourself and your own feelings.

You will thus be able to act and talk quite freely and naturally without being worried in the slightest by the presence of the others.

If you should begin to think about yourself or any negative thought, you will immediately shift your attention back to your conversation and you will no longer experience the slightest nervousness, discomfort, or uneasiness.

Anxiety

Relaxation will give you that peace of mind and inner tranquillity which will enable you to cope with the tensions and stresses of every-day living.

You will be able to adjust yourself to your environment even though you may not be able to change it.

You will be able to tolerate the persons, places or things that used to disturb and annoy you.

You can do everything better when you are relaxed, whether it be physical, mental or emotional.

You can and will control your entire body with your subconscious mind. Imagine controlling the muscles of your tongue, and you won't be saying things you will be sorry for in the future.

Relaxation will give you the courage and confidence that you need to take the T out of the word *can't* and find out that you can and that you will. Want it to happen; expect it to happen; and it will happen.

You are steadily losing your desire to be anxious. You are steadily increasing your desire to remove all emotional discomforts and become a completely empowered person.

As each of your worries is eliminated, it will not be replaced by another.

Pain and Healing

As you relax more and more, in hypnosis and self-hypnosis, the relaxation causes all the muscles and nerves in the affected area to become completely relaxed, thus relieving the symptom and causing the pain to disappear. As you become more and more relaxed in every way, you return to normal functioning and your body feels completely comfortable and free from all discomfort.

You are becoming desensitized in the various parts of your body where you have been complaining of pain. You will now find yourself recovering rapidly, with the healing process being greatly facilitated due to our recruitment of nature's healing forces. Natural-ly, the pain will not stop all at once, but you will find it lessening substantially each and every day. Any time you feel particularly uncomfortable, and this may happen for a few days, you will merely make yourself comfortable, close your eyes, and say 20, 20, 20. The act of counting is a post-hypnotic suggestion intended to relieve the discomfort. The act of counting will cause you to become desensi-tized and anesthetized in those parts of the body where you are uncomfortable and you will rapidly resume a relaxed and comfort-able condition. You will also find yourself pleasantly hungry at meal-times and will be able to eat well and hold your food down satisfactorily. (This latter suggestion was given if there is nausea.) You are steadily losing your desire for pain and discomfort.

Feel yourself becoming a loving and forgiving person. Consider love as an end in itself. Express your desire to achieve a thorough mental house cleaning…use positive words and positive thoughts to become a loving, forgiving person.

Imagine the illness or pain bothering you. Focus your healing energies. Quickly erase this image of your illness and see yourself as being completely cured. Feel the freedom and happiness of being in perfect health. Hold on to this image, linger over it, enjoy it, and know that you deserve it. Know that now in this healthy state you are fully in tune with nature's intentions for you.

Every day, in every way you are getting better, better, and better. Negative thoughts and negative suggestions have no influence over you at any mind level.

Visual Imagery

Visual imagery is also called creative visualization, guided imagery, or seeing with the mind's eye. This technique is useful in that it makes use of the mind's eye to picture positive actions and positive results; you can point it in the direction in which you want your life to go.

About 70 percent of us have a fairly easy time with visualization. The 30 percent who find this approach more difficult can still develop and strengthen their inner vision with practice. Mental images can be experienced as colorful mental movies, feelings or vibrations, black and white pictures, and images that are cloudy and are incomplete.

Hypnosis is one of the oldest techniques in psychology that use visualization. Using imagery indirectly to suggest relaxation signals your inner mind that it's time to settle down. Use of the past tense assumes that the response has been given. Since you receive the suggestion in the context of its having already been accomplished, you assume that it has, and therefore it is.

When a state of physiological relaxation has been established, simply visualize a pleasant, natural scene such as a little brook in a meadow or whatever occurs to you. Spend time and enjoy the scene so that you begin to experience the calming effect both of the fantasy and of holding it in the mind.

These various visualizations act to train the mind. We have already seen how they can be used in hypnotic induction techniques. Once you master this technique, you can create your own "mental movies" to remove habits and phobias, improve your immune system, and slow down the aging process.

The following scene should be practiced to train your subconscious to utilize your subconscious to create impressions suggesting relaxation and peace:

You are in a vast meadow with a huge expanse of blue sky above you. It is early spring. Smell the freshness in the air. In the distance you can see snow-covered mountains like the Alps or Himalayas. The meadow is green and covered with white daisies and other wildflowers. You wish to scale the mountain tops. You take an air pump and place the rubber hose in your mouth. You begin pumping your body with air, filling up like a balloon. The light, dry air inside your body gives you a sensation of weightlessness. You begin to float up into the blue sky. You are approaching the mountain peaks. It is getting colder as the altitude increases. The cold causes the air inside you to contract. You begin to descend, landing on the ridge of the mountain. It is freezing cold. The wind is blowing bitterly. With your back to the sheer side of the mountain, you inch your way along the ledge, snow blowing in your face.

You come to a pass. On the other side of the pass is another world. You cross the threshold and find yourself in an orchard of peaches. It is warm, like summer. There are fountains and marble statutes. Passing through the orchard, you come to a long flight of stone stairs leading to a rock palace. You walk up the steps and into the temple, finding yourself in a large stone chamber. There before you is a teak table on which is a stack of piping hot pancakes covered with butter and syrup. Next to them is a pitcher of milk. You begin eating the pancakes, washing them down with the milk. You are starved! They taste delicious and you eat and eat, shoveling the food down.

Suddenly a gong rings. It echoes throughout the chamber. A sliding stone panel opens and an ancient man with a long white beard enters, bearing a frothing glass of pink liquid. It is an ancient yeast drink, a health-food drink. He gives it to you and you drink. The yeast inside your stomach makes you feel lighter and lighter. The light, wet bubbles inside you make you feel airy as a feather. You float along the stone floor as if there were no gravity.

You glide along the floor, out the temple arch, down the steps, and to a river. You float like an innertube in the river to the very point where you entered the orchard. You are once again at the pass.

Youthing Imagery

For this next exercise you will need two photographs of yourself. One should be of you at a much younger age when you were healthy and vigorous. The second photo is to be a very recent one.

While in hypnosis, using one of the induction techniques already presented, concentrate on the picture of yourself at a younger age. Visualize your body (a particular part or organ) undergoing a change to re-create this youth in your current body. Do this for at least 10 minutes.

Now switch to the more recent photograph and repeat this procedure. Imagine an actual positive youthing change taking place in your body. Practice this exercise daily and change your focus to a different part of your body every seven days.

These next exercises require you to do some time traveling. Work on these one at a time, first placing yourself in self-hypnosis by playing your tape.

- Imagine the most significant change you will make in your life after age 75.

- Visualize where you will be living and who your friends are when you are 85.

- See yourself celebrating your 95th birthday.

- See yourself doing your favorite exercise or workout regimen at age 100.

- Focus on your greatest accomplishment at age 110.

- Describe in detail what your life will be like in the year 2025, 2045.

- Think about which part of your life will be more interesting and more fulfilled in 30 years, 50 years.

- Decide what age (at least 120) you will live to reach in a healthy and optimistic manner.

The purpose of these exercises is to program positive, longevity-boosting, and health-affirming paths to replace any negative images you may currently hold about your future. By seeing yourself as energetic, active, and healthy, you are slowing down the aging process. If you see a negative image about aging, say to yourself, "That doesn't apply to me, because I am programming my subconscious to initiate my youthing regimen now."

Cleansing

Before I present the last, and most important script, a discussion of hypnotic energy cleansing needs to be presented. This concept may sound strange and New Age, but understand that it was discovered and developed by me back in 1977 and is the main technique I utilize in my Los Angeles office. There are thousands of empowered souls throughout the world who will testify to its effectiveness. In fact, many have discussed their experiences on national television, radio, and in print.

In simple terms, cleansing is the introduction of the patient's subconscious mind to its perfect energy counterpart—the higher self or superconscious mind. I also refer to this as a superconscious mind tap.

Since the superconscious mind is perfect, and since neither the subconscious nor superconscious' energy levels can ever be lowered, this introduction has only two possible outcomes. Either nothing occurs (in which case I refer to this as "plateauing"), or the quality of the subconscious' energy level is raised.

When the second option is accomplished, the term "major breakthrough" is applied. Any issues or physical symptoms (aging signs, for example) that are reflected by the previous compromised and lower level of the subconscious are effectively resolved. Since the subconscious can never revert back to a lowered energy level once a major breakthrough is accomplished, this results in a permanent positive change in the patient.

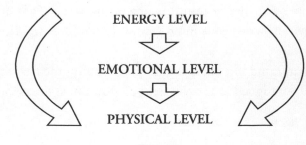

ENERGY LEVEL

EMOTIONAL LEVEL

PHYSICAL LEVEL

Figure 1
Cleansing

You will note that the arrows in Figure 1 always flow down from the energy level to the physical, but not in the reverse direction. Also observe that the energy level can change the physical level directly without having to use the emotional level as an intermediary. An example of this latter condition would be the removal of psychosomatic pain or a headache.

Raising energy levels eventually results in emotional and physical changes that ultimately slow down the aging process and accelerate the youthing mechanism. This process mostly takes place during our REM cycle at night. Since we spend approximately three hours each night in REM, and since our defense mechanism (the part of our mind that attempts to prevent any change occurring) cannot function during this time, this is a perfect opportunity for cleansing to manifest itself.

Ninety-eight percent of my therapy and a patient's youthing occurs during this REM phase. Each minute we spend in alpha (REM) is equivalent to at least three or four Earth minutes. We therefore receive the equivalent of up to 9 to 12 hours of cleansing each night. Is it any wonder this approach works so well?

There are three levels of manifestation of an issue. First, there is the physical level. Next comes the emotional level. Finally we have the energy level. The energy level controls the emotional level, which in turn affects the physical level. The only level I really concern myself with (and you should also take this approach) is the energy level. This level is reached best during the REM cycle, since the conscious mind proper (beta or analytical mind) is not in the way as it is during our waking day. This conscious mind cannot function at any time during our sleep cycle.

Keeping in mind this background, practice with the next script, as it is specifically designed to use cleansing to slow down the aging process.

Slowing Down the Aging Process

Now listen very carefully. I want you to imagine a bright white light coming down from above and entering the top of your head, filling your entire body. See it, feel it, and it becomes reality. Now imagine an aura of pure white light emanating from your heart region, again surrounding your entire body, protecting you. See it, feel it, and it becomes reality. Now only your higher self, masters and guides, and highly evolved loving entities who mean you well will be able to influence you during this or any other hypnotic session. You are totally protected by this aura of pure white light.

In a few moments I am going to count from 1 to 20. As I do so you will feel yourself rising up to the superconscious mind level where you will be able to receive experiences and information from your higher self. Number 1, rising up. 2, 3, 4, rising higher. 5, 6, 7, letting information flow. 8, 9, 10, you are halfway there. 11, 12, 13, feeling yourself rising even higher. 14, 15, 16, almost there. 17, 18, 19, number 20, you are there. Take a moment and orient yourself to the superconscious mind level.

PLAY NEW AGE MUSIC FOR 1 MINUTE

You are now in a deep hypnotic trance, and from this level you can improve the immune system of your physical body and slow down the process of aging. You are in complete control and able to access the limitless power of your superconscious mind. I want you to be open and flow with this experience. You are always protected by the white light.

At this time, I would like you to ask your higher self to facilitate step-by-step the raising of the frequency of your soul's energy. By doing this you will effect an energy cleansing that will bring about an emotional cleansing and an increase in all levels of the physical body's immune system. You are now slowing down the body's aging process. Do this now.

PLAY NEW AGE MUSIC FOR 3 MINUTES

Now, I would like you to allow this natural healing energy to spread throughout your entire physical body. Mentally picture yourself as you currently look and keep this image focused. Your body will now decelerate the normal process of aging. Your immune system will improve and resist diseases. Your adrenal glands will produce more and more DHEA-S hormone to bring about these desired results. Do this now.

PLAY NEW AGE MUSIC FOR 4 MINUTES

You have done very well. Now I want you to further open up the channels of communication by removing any obstacles and allowing yourself to receive information and experiences that will directly improve your ability to slow down the aging process and to help improve your present lifetime. Allow yourself to receive more advanced and more specific information from your higher self to raise the quality of your subconscious energy. Mentally picture yourself as you looked twenty years ago or longer. Keep this image focused. Your body will now slow down and even reverse the aging process to accomplish this. Do this now.

PLAY NEW AGE MUSIC FOR 4 MINUTES

All right now. Sleep now and rest. You did very, very well. Listen very carefully. I'm going to count forward now from 1 to 5. When I reach the count of 5, you will be back in the present. You will be able to remember everything you experienced and re-experienced. You'll feel very relaxed, refreshed, and you'll be able to do whatever you have planned for the rest of the day or evening. You'll feel very positive about what you've just experienced and very motivated about your confidence and ability to play this tape again to experience your higher self. All right now. 1, very, very deep. 2, you're getting a little bit lighter. 3, you're getting much, much lighter. 4, very, very light. 5, awaken. Wide awake and refreshed."

If you prefer professionally recorded tapes, simply contact Llewellyn or my office and I would be happy to send you a list of tapes recorded by me. A complete list of hypnotic aids and other helpful hints to assist you in making your own self-hypnosis tapes are given in my book, *New Age Hypnosis* (Llewellyn, 1998).

When we relax the mind and body with self-hypnosis, stress is automatically eliminated. Without stress there can be no real aging. The most natural and easy experience anyone can have is that of self-hypnosis. It is only because our waking state (beta) life is so encumbered with stress that we need to use alpha techniques.

Using the mind to consciously control the body is not a new idea. Eastern yogis, martial artists, and philosophers have been doing it for centuries. If you consciously control your thoughts and direct your subconscious mind in more tranquil directions, you can perceptibly influence heartbeat and blood pressure, and reduce stress and markedly slow down the aging process.

Using natural self-hypnosis will nourish both your mind and body. It is like being born. There is no better healer than positive thought to dissipate the ills of the body. Your subconscious mind is the key to healing, regeneration, and a healthy glow. If you want to experience youthing, then think young and you will effectively slow down the aging process. As Bob Dylan so aptly stated, "He who isn't being born is busy dying."

For those of you who seek the services of a qualified professional, there are detailed instructions in *New Age Hypnosis*. Here is a list of the types of health practitioners available today:

- A psychiatrist, or M.D. licensed by the state and able to prescribe drugs.

- A psychologist, a doctor of philosophy (Ph.D.) in psychology licensed by the state to help without prescribing drugs.

- A licensed clinical social worker (LCSW) with a master's degree in social work, usually affiliated with a community agency.

- A marriage, child, and family counselor, also licensed and with a master of arts (M.A.) or a master of science (M.S.) degree in a counseling field.

- An educational psychologist, licensed with a master's degree and experience working with children in schools.

All of these professionals are required to have at least 3,000 hours of supervised experience and pass tests to get their state licenses. As an alternative to those above, you might consult with:

- Clergy who do counseling under the auspices of a religious organization.

- Holistic practitioners, nutritionists, "counselors" and friends who may not be licensed, but who offer the potential of help through their unique approaches.

Always remember that the practice of cleansing and youthing techniques by professionals and patients alike can bring not only a larger view of inner and outer realities, but an increase in one's ecological and cosmic awareness. This can increase our physical longevity and bring into consciousness a realization that we and the universe are one. Thus, anything the individual does in this respect will come back to him/her.[2]

---

2   B. Goldberg, *Soul Healing* (St. Paul: Llewellyn, 1997).

14

CASE HISTORIES

The case histories in this chapter demonstrate that aging does not have to be characterized by the presence of chronic diseases such as heart disease, cancer, and arthritis. The development and severity of these diseases of aging is directly related to genetics and lifestyle. The other factor in combating aging, consciousness, has already been discussed in chapter 7.

Michelangelo, who painted the Sistine Chapel ceiling, was still painting at 88.

You cannot change your genetic heritage. If you were blessed with parents and grandparents who lived into their 80s or 90s or older, and who were relatively free of these chronic diseases, then you are most fortunate. However, a history of these relatives dying before the age of 60 from heart disease or cancer is a far less desirable heritage.

A positive genetic factor doesn't assure your longevity, but it adds to your potential. We can and should control our lifestyle. This is the most important consideration (along with consciousness raising), as I've discussed in the previous chapters.

The typical, frail elderly people you see have probably been dependent on others for their care for years. Most of their days are spent sitting or lying down. They often require assistance just to get out of a chair. Walking for many of them is usually impossible without the assistance of a cane or walker.

I have already explained why this occurs. Their muscle tissue is being replaced by fat, so they are weaker and more prone to heart disease and other chronic illnesses. The cases discussed here will illustrate the premise that the debilitation seen in many elderly is not a necessary or normal component of the aging process.

Before I present these case histories, let me comment on the late George Burns. George was born on January 20, 1896. He always expected to live to be 100, and did. Although he finally succumbed to Father Time, he did reach the century mark and left his mark on the world as an example of positive thinking.

George Burns was a family man. His career in vaudeville, radio, television, feature films, and night clubs covered over 75 years! Always an active man in his professional and personal life, he never lost his sense of humor. When asked to define old age he once wrote, "You'll know you're old . . . when you're still chasing women but can't remember why; when you stoop to tie your shoelaces and ask yourself, "What else can I do while I'm down here?"

George Burns never believed in retirement. He didn't work for so many years because he needed the money, he simply enjoyed his work. His comments on retirement reflect the theme of this book:

"To me the biggest danger of retirement is what it can do to your attitude. When you have all that time on our hands, you think old, you act old."[1]

"I will never retire! I firmly believe that you should keep working as long as you can. And if you can't, try to find something that will interest you. Keep your mind and body active. Remember, you can't help getting older, but you don't have to get old."[2]

---

1   G. Burns, *How to Live to Be 100 or More* (New York: G. P. Putnam's Sons, 1983), p. 131.
2   Ibid, p. 138.

I Practice What I Preach

In my previous books and scientific articles, I have always made it a policy to exclude as an example my own personal experiences with self-hypnosis and other regimens recommended in the books. Call it the objective scientist and clinician in me, but I intentionally refrained from injecting my own clinical use of these techniques into my writing.

I decided to break this pattern in this book for several reasons. For one, I have been using the techniques, especially self-hypnosis, for 30 years, and quite simply don't look my chronological age. As a "baby boomer," born on November 18, 1948, most people who meet me assume I'm in my early thirties. In fact, one Los Angeles physician accused me of lying about my age. He assumed I was trying to exaggerate my age to impress him, and he actually carded me!

My experience with youthing goes back over 30 years. People have always described me as a "gee whiz" idealist and highly motivated young man. Just last week I attended a cocktail party in Los Angeles, and a man I was speaking with disagreed intensely with my opinion about conventional medicine.

This man was a physician and 41 years old. He presented himself as overweight, sluggish, depressed, and frustrated in general. My alternative medicine emphasis and use of hypnosis bothered him greatly. He finally said to me, "When you reach my age, you will learn the truth about the value of modern medicine."

I informed him kindly that I was old enough to be his older brother and that if he was a model of what conventional medicine can do for the aging process, I'd take a rain check.

When I was in college I developed a relaxation technique that greatly improved my concentration, memory, and studying efficiency. As I had to work my way through college and dental school, this was an absolute necessity.

What I didn't realize at the time was that I was practicing self-hypnosis. As I have continued using this technique through the years (now 30 years later) I have noticed the difference it has made in my life.

I can play tennis, run, go parasailing, and participate in all of the sports I did as a teenager with equal—if not superior—agility and stamina. As a youth I was an excellent athlete, but had to curtail my endeavors with my entrance into college and dental school.

My last, and all previous EKGs were quite normal, and the results of my most recent cholesterol tests showed that my total cholesterol was 138 mg LDL (less than 200 is recommended) and my HDL cholesterol ratio was 2.8 (less than 4.5 is recommended). I am 5 feet 6 inches tall and weigh 130 pounds, five pounds less than in my college years in the late 1960s.

My reason for going into this personal history is to document the fact that I practice what I preach and am the beneficiary of the youthing program I expound. Too often we see weight reduction "experts" who are overweight and another example of "do what I say and not what I do."

I am not the exception, but the rule. Back in August of 1973 I was just about to enter my senior year at dental school. One particular Sunday I went sky diving. My girlfriend, a nursing student at the time, accompanied me, and was not excited about me jumping out of a Cessna 180 airplane at 2,900 feet.

She warned me that this exercise, assuming I survived, would age me significantly. Well, I experienced the most wonderful and exhilarating 90 seconds or so descent imaginable. I lived to tell about it, and contrary to the concern of my young lady friend, it didn't age me a bit.

Polly

Polly was one of my hypnosis patients, early in my career, back in 1977. This was shortly after I developed the superconscious mind tap or cleansing technique with self-hypnosis (discussed in chapter 13). She was 52 years *old* in 1977, with a history of arthritis, high blood pressure, high cholesterol counts, depression, smoking, and she was 50 pounds overweight.

In addition, Polly never exercised and had precancerous lesions diagnosed on her skin and breasts. There was a high probability of the lesions turning cancerous. Genetics was not on Polly's side; her father died of a stroke at age 54 (he had three heart attacks previously); her mother developed skin cancer, and died of breast cancer at age 56.

I worked with Polly on cleansing and youthing. She achieved only a light hypnotic trance level. Deeper levels of hypnosis are not necessary for cleansing to be effective, and this information greatly relieved her.

Polly expressed concern that her 21-year-old daughter would end up like her. Her daughter Carol was somewhat overweight and exhibited depression. I didn't work with Carol, as she was away at school. A few months later Polly moved to the Midwest and did not communicate with me again until June of 1996.

Polly apparently followed my career. She read my books and saw my televised interviews on Oprah, Donahue, CNN, Joan Rivers, Regis and Kathie Lee, and other shows. Having taken an executive position with a Midwest company (which fortunately did not have a mandatory age 65 retirement policy), Polly was kept pretty busy.

She was scheduled to go to Los Angeles for a business conference, and a synchronistic event occurred. Just prior to her leaving, she saw my interview on Leeza and decided to look me up while out here on the Coast.

You can imagine my surprise when she called. I invited her over to the office for a chat and was amazed at what I observed. This now 71-year-*young* woman was at least 50 pounds thinner than our previous meeting. She no longer smoked, exercised daily, no longer suffered from arthritis, appeared free of depression, and had an acceptable cholesterol count and blood pressure reading. Most important to her, there were no signs of cancer.

Our conversation was one of the most enjoyable I have had in years. The fact that this rather complex history of chronic aging disorders was reversed, and a 71-year-young former patient, who looked twenty years younger, presented herself to me after the synchronicity of viewing me on an NBC daytime talk show, only added to the testimony of the power of consciousness expansion.

One final note about this case had to do with Carol. In 1982 Polly purchased my superconscious mind self-hypnosis tape for her daughter as a Christmas present. Carol used this cassette diligently and followed in her mother's footsteps therapeutically.

Carol lost 25 pounds, became active and now, at age 40 (Polly showed me a recent photo of her, along with one when Carol was 21), had the appearance of a woman in her late twenties. All this was stimulated by her own consciousness without ever seeing me, just by playing my tape.

Both Carol and Polly have a long and productive life ahead of them. Their relationship markedly improved after Carol's cleansing experiences. It puts a new twist on the old saying, "the family that 'youths' together stays together."

Jerome

In 1985 a 58-year-old trial lawyer named Jerome came to see me. He didn't have a particularly high opinion of hypnosis, but my therapy was highly recommended by one of his colleagues, whose wife I had successfully empowered the previous year.

Jerome lived a high-pressure lifestyle. His practice was very demanding and suited his highly skeptical, arrogant, and argumentative personality. He smoked two packs a day, was 35 pounds overweight, had Type II insomnia, and very poor muscular strength.

In short, Jerome was aging rapidly. His history of crash diets, diet pills, nicotine gum, too much television, and high-calorie dinners out were taking its toll. As a divorced man, Jerome also longed for female companionship.

It was not easy to work with him. The combination of his argumentativeness and arrogance, coupled with anger at his degenerating body, tested even my patience. Fortunately, cleansing techniques were quickly successful and Jerome acknowledged this positive feedback as the light at the end of the tunnel.

Explaining cleansing techniques to him was no easy chore. It wasn't that Jerome lacked the intellectual capacity to comprehend the energy-to-emotion-to-physical paradigm, his skepticism simply played into his natural defense mechanism's resistance to change.

Jerome was a conscientious man and kept in touch with me for several months following his relatively short therapy. He reported losing about 15 pounds, giving up smoking, and generally having more energy. A business trip to Los Angeles in 1995 prompted another visit with me.

Jerome called me when he arrived in Los Angeles to thank me for his "new life." I agreed to meet him for coffee one evening to see how his new life was going. What I saw was an enthusiastic, trim, and vigorous man who looked like he was in his early fifties.

This trial lawyer was 68 when we met again. He informed me how he had taken up coin collecting and purchased a German Shepherd dog. Jerome had never owned a pet before.

My query concerning his social life revealed that my former patient was living with his 40-year-young girlfriend. His youthing results were nothing short of astounding. He was no longer argumentative (at least when he was not in court) and the only bone of contention was his awarding far too much credit for his growth on me. At least 98 percent of his youthing resulted from his actions. I merely trained him.

Emma

The last case concerns a 75-year-old woman named Emma. She had seen me on the Joan Rivers Show in May of 1990 and immediately purchased my first book, *Past Lives—Future Lives*.

She was so intrigued with my work that she flew from Florida to Los Angeles on relatively short notice to begin her youthing training. Emma looked her age and more when I saw her in 1990. This well-meaning soul had arthritis, spastic colitis, high blood pressure, and very little energy.

Emma suffered from Types I, II, and III insomnia, and was mildly depressed. Her motivation was excellent though, and she expressed a great willingness to work on the youthing regimen.

After cleansing trainings were completed, I made various other recommendations for diet and exercise. She promised to follow through on these regimens and contact me at some future time to report on her progress.

In 1995 Emma returned to Los Angeles on a vacation with several of her friends. This now eighty-one-year-young woman looked twenty years younger than her chronological age. She no longer suffered from arthritis, colitis, or insomnia. Emma's blood pressure was normal and she had plenty of energy.

I met her friends; their only complaint concerning Emma was that she was impossible to keep up with, even on a slow day. Emma's youthing was and is successful because of her efforts and the fact that these simple methods really do work.

CONCLUSION

According to the National Institute of Aging, the number of people age 58 and older is growing rapidly and is soon expected to make up almost 25 percent of the older population (over 65), with women outnumbering men 5 to 2.

We, as a society, are striving not just to live longer, but to live better. We seek a way to avoid the chronic diseases, encroaching fatigue, and degrading changes that seem to characterize old age. As a nation, we are searching to find what we can do to make our lives better, extend our most healthy, vibrant, active years, and shorten the time of weakness and failing health. We are a people ripe and ready to empower ourselves and apply natural youthing techniques.

Biochemical gerontologist Dr. Denham Harman stated, "A major objective now and in the future should be maximizing health and well-being...so as to make life worth living for as long as possible. This will require a more careful application of preventive medicine."[1] More and more studies show how we can slow—and, in some cases, even reverse the cellular processes of decay and aging. For example, the NIA budget is well over 200 million dollars and the agency funds over 700 research projects. More than 34 medical journals are devoted to aging and aging prevention, and in the United States there are over a dozen scientific institutions devoted solely to anti-aging research and study.

---

1   D. Harman, op. cit.

Science has made great strides forward in the understanding of just what aging is, how it works, and—most important of all—what we can do about it. We can reduce the diseases of aging and prolong our health and vital years. In short, we are now able to look younger and live longer naturally.

Over 85 percent of the debilitating illnesses of old age result from only a handful of diseases—cancer, coronary artery disease, stroke, diabetes, kidney failure, obstructive lung disease, pneumonia, and influenza. Heart disease, all by itself, accounts for fully one out of every two deaths of older Americans, and high blood pressure directly causes or contributes to 15 percent of all deaths. We now can control even these pathologies by our lifestyle.

Dr. Peter Greenwald, director of Cancer Prevention and Control at the National Cancer Institute, says that 80 percent of cancer cases are linked to how we live our lives—so [cancer] can be controlled.[2] Dr. Edward Schneider, Dean of USC's Gerontology Center, says, "Adding life to years, not just years to life, is the goal of aging research."[3] By the simple act of knowing how to eat, exercise, and live your life so you can lower your risk for these diseases of aging (and incorporating this knowledge into your lifestyle), you automatically improve your chances of avoiding the causes of premature aging, debility, and death.

The most important message of this book is to keep a young mind and healthy body. Enthusiasm, meeting people, having plans, and keeping busy is what I mean by a young mind. Many older people simply give up and decide that their life is over. I suggest you look to the future, a long future.

Living in the past is a sign of depression. Old memories are fine, but you've still got time to make new memories. When people get a little older they are frightened to make a change in their lives. It's easier to stay in that same safe rut. To me that challenge is what keeps us alive and "in the flow."

---

2   P. Greenwald, *Cancer, Diet and Nutrition: A Comprehensive Sourcebook* (Chicago: Marquis Who's Who Professional Publishing Division, 1985).

3   E. Schneider, *Questions About the Beginning of Life* (Minneapolis: Augsburg Pub. House, 1985).

Just because you're chronologically old doesn't mean you can't lead a full, vigorous, and active life. Open your mind to it, don't just sit there—do things. The possibilities are endless. Try doing something nice for somebody who doesn't expect it. You'll be surprised how good you'll feel.

Funerals are another ritual to keep away from. I realize how society has used guilt to program us to attend this charade of emotional confabulation. If you really respect and appreciate someone, show it to them during their life. Don't wait until it's too late. Funeral services tend to focus our minds on our own mortality, and that is a guaranteed formula for depression.

The late George Burns said it best when he described his feelings about funerals:

"To me, funerals are like bad movies. They last too long, they're overacted, and the ending is predictable. Another thing I don't understand about funerals: all the mourners show up in their somber clothes—black veils, black ties, black handkerchiefs. The deceased is the only one wearing a beige suit with a powder-blue shirt and a matching polka-dot tie. He looks great and we all look pathetic."[4]

Well-Span

I like to call living an extended and quality life "well-span" rather than life span. Living the longest possible life and being energetic, fully alert, and radiantly alive is definitely within our grasp. You can forget about the stereotype of the doddering, feeble-minded man or woman with minimally functioning faculties. Following these recommendations will help you keep joy in your heart, a sparkle in your eyes, and a spring in your step for many decades to come.

To accomplish this you must avoid worry, stress and tension. Remember, worry leads to stress, and stress leads to tension. Former Secretary of Health, Education, and Welfare Joseph A. Califano, Jr.,

---

4 Burns, op. cit., p. 131.

testified before the United States Senate and stated, "67% of all disease and premature death is preventable."[5] Now doesn't that reduce your worrying (stress and tension)?

The Ethics of Longevity

One controversial aspect of extending our life expectancy, especially with genetic research, is that it is tantamount to advocating eugenics. Those that object to this form of progress most likely assume the world would be overpopulated with medically compromised men and women who simply don't want to die.

A careful evaluation of the facts presented in *Look Younger, Live Longer* shows that we will have an increase in the number of elderly men and women like none who have preceded them, living for many years in the vigorous possession of their powers. This, I believe, will convince even the most cynical of people that more and more people will wish this outcome for themselves and for those they love, and the arguments for preventing others from taking advantage of this knowledge to this end will grow steadily weaker and less frequent.

Another factor to consider is how we spend our lives. In our early years we are directed in our development by others. They educate us and assist us in our preparation to become creative and productive citizens. When we have reached the stage where we are considered educated, mature, ready for adulthood, we marry and begin to have children and rear the next generation—whose education and development we then undertake as our major responsibility.

We make many sacrifices during these parenting years—to earn a living, pay the rent, and otherwise provide for our family. During these "best years of our lives" we postpone many pleasures, activities, and ambitions, but do we do this just so our children can repeat this cycle?

---

5   J. A. Califano, *America's Health Care Revolution: Who Lives? Who Dies? Who Pays?* (New York: Random House, 1986).

When the children have left the nest and are launched in their own lives, we finally have time to indulge ourselves in what we want and like to do. By that time we come to the realization that our health and vigor are compromised. Just when we could best make use of a generous stretch of time, we become acutely aware of how little time is left to us—and that awareness colors everything we think and do. We are depressed by the thought that perhaps we have wasted our lives. Epicurus said it best when he commented that most people spend their lives preparing for death.

There is a principle in genetics that states that most mutations are harmful and only a small percent actually contribute to positive evolution. I feel that we could create our own mutations that would result in far less human misery. We could actually eliminate aging and premature death!

However, this is a book on natural methods of youthing, so I will forego eugenic arguments. Think what the world would be like with an average well-span of 120 years or more. These new and productive citizens could resynthesize, in collaboration with similar long-livers, whole new systems of thought, bringing together mathematics, physics, astronomy, cosmology, geology, meteorology, chemistry, paleontology, archeology, biology, psychology, medicine, anthropology, sociology, economics, history, politics, art, literature, drama, poetry, music, theology, law, philosophy—the entire catalogue of human disciplines, plus others yet to be created.

We as a species could then finally become all that we could be, and the universe would most likely be better off for it. Think of the great minds that are lost to society due to premature death. I do feel that there is purpose in the universe. Where do we really fit into this design as a species or as individuals?

To be worthy of this longevity we must learn to be truly human. By this I refer to transcending our present selves in ways that will demand all the courage, compassion, imagination, good sense, and good cheer that we can muster. The mustering of those resources would, I think, be considerably enhanced by the addition of good years to good lives. We simply mustn't continue to repeat history's errors.

Final Thoughts

We can slow down, and in some cases reverse, many of the physiological and biochemical declines associated with the process of growing older. You will notice I omitted the term *aging* from the last statement. The research presented has shown that aging is mostly a state of mind.

To incorporate this youthing process in your well-span will require approximately one hour each day for exercise and self-hypnosis. Is that a lot to ask for qualitatively extending your life by 25 to 50 years? You do not have to disrupt your life to follow this suggested regimen.

The only requirement in youthing is a willingness to incorporate the very successful techniques and paradigms presented in this book. Natural life-extending procedures are no longer mere speculation. They do work. The question remains not if you can attain these most desirable goals, but when?

Death has, for the first time in history, lost its occult mystique. Stripped of its paralyzing mystery, death becomes merely a biological malfunction instead of a health process to be feared.

Life, not death, remains the mystery. My true purpose is to enhance life and belittle death by this demystification. Perhaps living to an age of 140, 160, or even 200 is not immortality. Who knows what geneticists and other scientists will develop by then to solve the riddle of why DNA's replication mechanism breaks down with time?

True immortality is a state of mind. Since our consciousness is the most important component of our being, let the wonders of the universe unfold before us. May we all become empowered in our most unusual journey through the labyrinth of consciousness and space.

Try these techniques and heed the advice given. I will look forward to hearing from you 75, 100, or 150 years from now.

BIBLIOGRAPHY

Adelan, Richard C., and Gary W. Britton. "The Impaired Capability for Biochemical Adapation During Aging." *BioScience,* October 1975.

Adler, William H. "Aging and Immune Function." *BioScience,* October 1975.

Alexander, C. N., H. M. Chandler, E. J. Langer, R. I. Newman, and J. L. Davies. "Transcendental Meditation, Mindfulness and Longevity: An Experimental Study with the Elderly." *Journal of Personal Social Psychology,* 57, 1989.

Anderson, J. W., and N. J. Gustafsson. "Type II Diabetes: Current Nutrition Management Concepts." *Geriatrics* 41, 1986.

Andres, Reubin. "The Normality of Aging: The Baltimore Longitudinal Study," summary presentation at NIA/GRC, Baltimore, October 1976.

Barrows, Charles H., Jr. "The Challenge-Mechanisms of Biological Aging," *Gerontologist,* Spring 1971.

_____. "Ecology of Aging and the Aging Process—Biological Parameters." *Gerontologist,* Summer 1968.

Batten, Mary. "Life Spans." *Science Digest,* February 1984.

Becker, Ernest. *The Denial of Death.* New York: The Free Press (Macmillan), 1973.

Behnke, John A., Caleb E. Finch, and Gairdner B. Moment (eds). *The Biology of Aging.* New York: Plenum Press, 1978.

Benet, Sula. *How to Live to Be 100: The Life-Style of the People of the Caucasus.* New York: Dial Press, 1976.

Beverly, E. Virginia. "Exploring the Many-Faceted Mysteries of Aging." *Geriatrics,* March 1975.

Bortz, Edward L. *Creative Aging.* New York: Macmillan, 1963.

Bortz, Walter M. II. "Disuse and Aging." *Journal of the American Medical Association* 248, No. 10, September 10, 1982.

Breslow, Lester. "Health Priorities and Quality Care Evidence from Alameda County" *Preventive Medicine: An International Journal Devoted to Prace and Theory,* January 1993.

Brody, Jane E. "Hope Grows for Vigorous Old Age." *New York Times,* October 2, 1984.

Brody, Harold, and Henryk M. Wisniewski. "Genetics of Human Aging." *Review of Biological Research in Aging,* 1983.

Brown, W. Ted. "Human Mutations Affecting Aging—A Review." *Mechanisms of Aging and Development.* Vol. 9, 1979.

Bullough, W. S. "Aging of Mammals." *Nature,* Vol. 299, 1971.

Burkitt, Dennis, et al. *Dietary Fibre, Fibre-depleted Foods and Disease.* London: Academic Press, 1975.

Burns, George. *How to Live to Be 100 or More.* New York: G. P. Putnam's Sons, 1983.

Butler, Robert N. "Medicine and Aging: An Assessment of Opportunities and Neglect," testimony before U.S. Senate Special Committee on Aging, October 13, 1976.

_____. *Why Survive? Being Old in America.* New York: Harper & Row, 1975.

Califano, J. A. *America's Health Care Revolution: Who Lives? Who Dies? Who Pays?* New York: Random House, 1986.

Campbell, D. T., and J. C. Stanley. *Experimental and Quasi-Experimental Designs for Research.* Chicago: Rand McNally, 1963.

Carrel, Alexis. *Voyage to Lourdes.* New York: Harper, 1950.

Cutler, Richard G. "Antioxidants, Aging and Longevity," in *Free Radicals in Biology*. Vol. 6 (W. A. Pryor, ed.). New York: Academic Press, 1983.

_____. "Evolution of Human Longevity and the Genetic Complexity Governing Aging Rate." *Proceedings of the National Academy of Sciences,* November 1975.

Davies, David. "A Shangri-la in Ecuador," *New Scientist,* February 1, 1973.

Dawson-Hughes, B., et al. "Dietary Calcium Intake and Bone Loss from the Spine in Healthy Postmenopausal Women." *American Journal of Clinical Nutrition* 46, 1987.

Daynes, R. A., et al. "Altered Regulation of IL-6 Production with Normal Aging: Possible Linkage to the Age-Associated Decline in Dehydroepiandrosterone and its Sulfated Derivative." *Journal of Immunology* 150 (12), 1993.

Denckla, W. Donner. "Is There a Biological Aging Clock?" Interview in *Anti-Aging News,* September 1981.

_____. "Searching for the 'Death' Hormone." Interview in *Anti-Aging News,* October 1981

_____. "A Time to Die." *Life Sciences,* Vol. 16, 1974.

Donahue, R. P., et al. "Central Obesity and Coronary Heart Disease in Men." *Lancet* 8537, 1987.

Dukas, Helen, and Banesh Hoffman, eds. *Albert Einstein: The Human Side.* Princeton: Princeton University Press, 1979.

Dunbar, Flanders. *Mind and Body Psychosomatic Medicine.* New York: Random House, 1955.

Dychtwald, K. *Age Wave.* Los Angeles: Jeremy P. Tarcher, 1989.

Eaton, S. Boyd, et al. *The Paleolithic Prescription: A Program of Diet & Exercise & a Design for Living.* New York: Harper-Row, 1989.

Fries, J. F. *Living Well: Taking Care of Your Health in the Middle and Later Years.* Reading, Mass.: Addison-Wesley Pub. Co., 1994.

Frolkis, V. V. "Regulation and Adaptation Processes in Aging." *The Main Problems of Soviet Gerontology,* Kiev, 1972.

Frolkis, V. V., et al. "The Hypothalamus in Aging." *Experimental Gerontology,* Vol. 7, 1972.

Fromm, E. "Altered States of Consciousness and Hypnosis: A Discussion." *International Journal of Clinical Experimental Hypnosis* 25, 1977.

Frontera, W. R., et al. "Strength Conditioning in Older Men: Skeletal Muscle Hypertrophy and Improved Function." *Journal of Applied Physiology* 64, 1988.

Gold, Michael. "The Cells That Would Not Die." *Science* 81, April 1981.

Goldberg, Bruce. "Hypnosis and the Immune Response." *International Journal of Psychosomatics,* 32(3), 1985.

_____. "Slowing Down the Aging Process Through the Use of Altered States of Consciousness: A Review of the Medical Literature." *Psychology—A Journal of Human Behavior,* 32(2), 1995.

_____. *Soul Healing.* St. Paul: Llewellyn, 1996.

_____. "The Treatment of Cancer Through Hypnosis." *Psychology—A Journal of Human Behavior,* 3(4), 1985.

Goldstein, Samuel. "Biological Aging: An Essentially Normal Process," *Journal of the American Medical Association,* December 23–30, 1974.

Gordon, N. F., and L. W. Gibbons. *The Cooper Clinic Cardiac Rehabilitation Program.* New York: Simon & Schuster, 1990.

Greenwald, Peter. *Cancer, Diet and Nutrition: A Comprehensive Sourcebook.* Chicago: Marquis Who's Who Professional Pub. Division, 1985.

Hagelin, J. S. "Is Consciousness the Unified Field? A Field Theorist's Perspective." *Modern Science and Vedic Science,* 1(1), 1987.

Harman, Denham. "Free Radical Theory on Aging: Dietary Implications." *American Journal of Clinical Nutrition,* August 1972.

Harrison, David E. "Experience with Developing Assays of Physiological Age," in *Biological Markers of Aging* (M. E. Reff and E. L. Schneider, eds.). Bethesda, Maryland: National Institutes of Health, 1982.

_____. "Must We Grow Old?" *Biology Digest,* February 1982.

Hayflick, Leonard. "The Biology of Human Aging." *American Journal of Medical Sciences* 265, 1973.

_____."Recent Advances in the Cell Biology of Aging." *Mechanisms of Aging and Development,* Vol. 14, 1980.

Henderson, E., et al. "Dehydropepiandrosterone (DHEA) and Synthetic DHEA Analogs are Modest Inhibitors of HIV-I IIIB Replication." *AIDS Reserach Human Retroviruses* 8 (5), 1992.

Hochschild, Richard. "Effect of Dimethylaminoethanol on the Life Span of Senile Male A/J Rats." *Experimental Gerontology,* Vol. 8, 1973.

Hopson, Janet L. Interview with Marian Diamond, *Psychology Today,* Nov. 1984.

James, William. *The Principles of Psychology.* New York: Henry Holt, 1890.

Jones, Hardin B. *Sensual Drugs: Deprivation and Rehabilitation of the Mind.* Boston: Cambridge University Press, 1976.

Kahn, Robert L. *Work and Health.* New York: Wiley, 1981.

Katcher, A., and Beck, A. *New Perspectives on Our Lives with Companion Animals.* Philadelphia: University of Pennsylvania Press, 1983.

Kestersnon, D. *Josh Billings.* New York: Twayne, 1973.

Kiecolt-Glaser, J. K., et al. "Psychosocial Enhancement of Immuncompetence in a Geriatric Population." *Health Psychology* 4, 1985.

Langer, Ellen. *Mindfullness.* Reading, Mass.: Addison-Wesley, 1989.

Larsson., L., et al. "Muscle Strength and Speed of Movement in Relation to Age and Muscle Morphology." *Journal of Applied Physiology* 46, 1979.

Leaf, Alexander. "The Aging Process: Lessons from Observations in Man." *Nutrition Review,* February 1988.

_____. "The Peaks of Old Age." *Observer Magazine,* Sept. 30, 1973.

_____. *Youth in Old Age.* New York: McGraw-Hill, 1975.

_____. "Where Life Begins at 100." *National Geographic,* Jan. 1973.

Loria, R. M., et al. "Immune Response Facilitation and Resistance to Virus and Bacterial Infections with Dehydroepiandrosterone (DHEA)." In *The Biologic Role of Dehydroepiandrosterone.* M. Kalimi, and W. Regelson, eds. New York: Walter de Gruyter 1990.

Luce, Gay. *Your Second Life.* New York: Delacorte Press, 1979.

Maranto, Gina. "Aging: Can We Slow the Inevitable?" *Discover,* December 1984.

Martin, G., et al. "Replicative Life Span of Cultivated Human Cells: Effect of Donor's Age, Tissue and Genotype." *Laboratory Investigation,* 1970, 23 (1).

Masters, Robert, and Jean Houston. *Listening to the Body.* New York: Delacorte press, 1978.

Miller, Judith K., Robert Bolla, and W. Donner Denckla. "Age-Associated Changes in Initiation of Ribonucleic Acid Synthesis in Isolated Rat Liver Nuclei," *Journal of Biochemistry,* Vol. 188, 1980.

Moment, Gairdner. "The Ponce de Leon Trail Today." *BioScience,* Oct. 1975.

Montagu, Ashley. *Growing Young.* New York: McGraw-Hill, 1981.

Moss, C. S. *Hypnosis in Perspective.* New York: Macmillan, 1965.

Najafi, Hassan, "Dr. Alexis Carrel and Tissue Culture." *Journal of the American Medical Association,* August 27, 1983.

National Institute on Aging. *Handbook for the Biology of Aging.* Washington: U.S. Govt. Printing Office, 1985.

_____. "With the Passage of Time: The Baltimore Longitudinal Study of Aging." *N.I.H.* Pub. No. 93–3685, 1985.

Neugarten, Bernice L., and Robert J. Havighurst (eds.). *Extending the Human Life Span: Social Policy and Social Ethics.* Washington: Superintendent of Documents, U.S. Printing Office, 1977.

Newsweek. "Can Aging Be Cured?" April 16, 1973.

Nikitin, V. N. "The Genetic Apparatus and Aging Processes." *The Main Problems of Soviet Gerontology,* 1972.

Orentreich, N., et al. "Age Changes and Sex Differences in Serum DHEA-S Concentrations Throughout Adulthood." *Journal of Clinical Endocrinological Metabolism,* 59, 551, 1984.

Ornstein, Robert, and Sobel, David. *The Healing Brain: Breakthrough Medical Discoveries About How the Brain Keeps Us Healthy.* New York: Simon & Schuster, 1987.

Ostlund, R. E. Jr., et al. "The Ratio of Waist-to-Hip Circumference, Plasma Insulin Level, and Glucose Intolerance as Independent Predictors of the HDL (sub 2) Cholesterol Level in Older Adults." *New England Journal of Medicine* 322, 1990.

Palmore, Erdman. "Predicting Longevirty: A New Method." *Normal Aging II: Reports from the Duke Longitudinal Study, 1970–1973.* Durham, North Carolina: Duke University Press, 1974.

Pashko, L. L., et al. "Inhibition of 7, 12-dimethylbenz (a) Anthracene-induced Skin Papilomas and Carcinomas by Dehydroepiandrosterone and 3-beta-methylandrost-5-en-17-one in Mice." *Cancer Research* 45(1) (1985): 164–66.

Pavlov, E. P., S. M. Harman, G.P. Chrousos, D.L. Loriaux, and M. R. Blackman. "Responses of Plasma Adrenocorticotropin, Cortisol, and Dehydroepiandrosterone to Ovine Corticotropin-releasing Hormone in Healthy Aging Men." *Journal of Clinical Endocrinological Metabolism,* 62, 767, 1986.

Pelletier, Kenneth R. *Longevity: Fulfilling Our Biological Potential.* New York: Delacorte Press/Seymour Lawrence, 1981.

_____. *Holistic Medicine: From Stress to Optimum Health.* New York: Delacorte Press/Seymour Lawrence, 1979.

Penfield, Wilder. *The Mystery of the Mind: A Critical Study of Consciousness and the Human Brain.* Princeton: Princeton University Press, 1975.

Presmen, Curtis, and the Editors of *Esquire. How a Man Ages.* New York: Ballantine Books, 1984.

Rasmussen, K. R., et al. "Effects of Dexamethasone and Dehydroepiandrosterone in Immunosupressed Rats Infected with Cryptosporidium Parvum." *Journal of Protozoology* 38(6) (1991): 1575–1595.

Regelson, William, and F. Marott Sinex (eds.). *Intervention in the Aging Process,* 2 vols. New York: Alan R. Liss, 1983.

Regelson, William, et al. "Hormonal Intervention: 'Buffer Hormones' or 'State Dependency.' The Role of Dehydroepiandrosterone (DHEA), Thyroid Hormone, Estrogen and Hyphosectomy in Aging." *Annals of New York Academy of Science* 521, 1988.

Riesberg, Barry. *Brain Failure: An Introduction to Current Concepts of Senility.* New York: The Free Press, 1981.

Rosenfield, Albert. "Aging Well Is the Best Revenge." *Gentleman's Quarterly,* March 1984.

_____. "Do You Want to Live to Be 120?" *Prime Time,* February 1980.

_____. "In Search of Youth." *Geo,* June 1982.

_____. "Interview-W. Donner Denckla," *Omni,* November 1981.

_____, (ed.), "Mind and Supermind: Expanding the Limits of Consciousness." Special section in *Saturday Review,* February 22, 1975.

Schock, Nathan, R. C. Greulich, et al. *Normal Human Aging.* Washington: U.S. Govt. Printing Office, 1984.

Schrauzer. "Selenium and Cancer: A Review," *Bioinorg. Chemistry.* 5, 1976.

Seals, D. M., et al. "Endurance Training in Older Men and Women, 1: Cardiovascular Responses to Exercise." *Journal of Applied Physiology* 57, 1984.

Shamberger, "Relationship of Selenium to Cancer. I. Inhibitory Effect of Selenium on Carcinogenesis" *Journal of the National Cancer Institute,* 44(4), April 1970.

Simonton, O. C., S. Matthews-Simonton, and J. L. Creighton. *Getting Well Again.* Los Angeles: Tarcher-St. Martins, 1978.

Simonton, O. C., S. Matthews-Simonton, and T. F. Sparks. "Psychological Intervention in the Treatment of Cancer." *Psychosomatics,* 21, 1980.

Sinex, F. Marott. "Genetic Mechanisms of Aging." *Journal of Gerontology,* July 1966.

Sprott, Richard L. *Age, Learning Ability and Intelligence.* New York: Van Nostrand Reinhold, 1980.

Stein, J. and L. J. Kleinsmith. "Chromosomal Proteins and Gene Regulation." *Scientific American,* February 1975.

Strehler, Bernard L. *Time, Cells and Aging.* New York: Academic Press, 1977.

Thomas, Lewis. "Medicine's New Role: Helping the Elderly to Stay Fit in Body, Mind and Spirit," *Discover,* December 1984.

Tierney, John. "The Aging Body." *Esquire,* May, 1982.

Truswell, A. S., et al. "Blood Pressure of Kung Bushmen in Northern Botswana." *American Heart Journal* 84, 1972.

Tuccille, Jerome. *Here Comes Immortality.* New York: Stein & Day, 1974.

Vaillant, George. *Adaptation of Life.* Boston: Little Brown, 1977.

Vidik, Andrus. Lectures on Gerontology, Vol. IA: *On Biology of Aging.* New York: Academic Press, 1982.

von Hahn, H. "The Regulation of Protein Synthesis in Aging Cell." *Experimental Gerontology,* October 1970.

Walford, Roy L. *The Immunologic Theory of Aging.* Baltimore: William & Wilkins, 1969.

_____. *Maximum Life Span.* New York: W. W. Norton, 1983.

Wallace, R. K., M. C. Dillbeck, E. Jacobe, and B. Harrington. "Effects of the TM and TM-Sidhi Program on the Aging Process." *International Journal of Neuroscience,* 16, 1982.

Watson, James D., and Francis H. C. Crick, "A Structure for Deoxyribose Nucleic Acid." *Nature,* April 25, 1953.

Webb, J. N. "Muscular Dystrophy and Muscle Cell Death in Normal Foetal Development." *Nature,* November 15, 1974.

Weil, A. *Spnataneous Healing.* New York: Alfred A. Knopf, 1995.

Whitten, Joan. "Cell Death During Early Morphogenesis: Parallels Between Insect Limb and Vertebrae Limb Development." *Science,* March 28, 1969.

Wigner, Eugene. *Physical Science and Human Values.* Princeton: Princeton University Press, 1947.

Winter, Ruth. *Ageless Aging.* New York: Crown Publishers, 1973.

INDEX

3   Ibid.

☾ LOOK FOR THE CRESCENT MOON

Llewellyn publishes hundreds of books on your favorite subjects! To get these exciting books, including the ones on the following pages, check your local bookstore or order them directly from Llewellyn.

ORDER BY PHONE

- Call toll-free within the U.S. and Canada, 1-800-THE MOON
- In Minnesota, call (612) 291-1970
- We accept VISA, MasterCard, and American Express

ORDER BY MAIL

- Send the full price of your order (MN residents add 7% sales tax) in U.S. funds, plus postage & handling to:

  Llewellyn Worldwide
  P.O. Box 64383, Dept. K–321–2
  St. Paul, MN 55164–0383, U.S.A.

POSTAGE AND HANDLING

(For the U.S., Canada, and Mexico)

- $4.00 for orders $15.00 and under
- $5.00 for orders over $15.00
- No charge for orders over $100.00

We ship UPS in the continental United States. We ship standard mail to P.O. boxes. Orders shipped to Alaska, Hawaii, The Virgin Islands, and Puerto Rico are sent first-class mail. Orders shipped to Canada and Mexico are sent surface mail.

International orders: Airmail—add freight equal to price of each book to the total price of order, plus $5.00 for each non-book item (audio tapes, etc.).

Surface mail—Add $1.00 per item.

Allow 4–6 weeks for delivery on all orders.
Postage and handling rates subject to change.

DISCOUNTS

We offer a 20 percent discount to group leaders or agents. You must order a minimum of 5 copies of the same book to get our special quantity price.

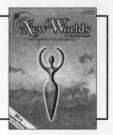
Visit our website at www.llewellyn.com for more information.

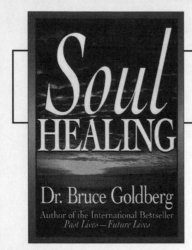

SOUL HEALING
Dr. Bruce Goldberg

George: overcame lung cancer and a life of smoking through hypnotic programming.

Mary: tripled her immune system's response to AIDS with the help of age progression.

Now you, too, can learn to raise the vibrational rate of your soul (or subconscious mind) to stimulate your body's own natural healing processes. Explore several natural approaches to healing that include past life regression and future life progression, hypnotherapy, soulmates, angelic healing, near-death experiences, shamanic healing, acupuncture, meditation, yoga, and the new physics.

The miracle of healing comes from within. After reading *Soul Healing*, you will never view your life and the universe in the same way again.

1-56718-317-4, 6 x 9, 304 pp., softcover   **$14.95**

THE SEARCH FOR GRACE
THE TRUE STORY OF MURDER & REINCARNATION

Dr. Bruce Goldberg

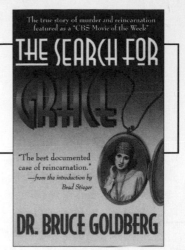

An unsolved murder mystery on the books since 1927…one modern woman's obsession with an abusive lover…and a karmic journey that winds through a maze of past lives—all of these unite into the *best*-documented case of reincarnation in the Western world.

The Search for Grace is the true story of Ivy, a 26-year-old pharmacist who sought the help of Dr. Bruce Goldberg to put a stop to her inexplainable attraction to John, her physically and psychologically abusive boyfriend. Under hypnosis, she discovered that John had been her lover—and her murderer—in 20 of her 46 past lives.

When Ivy recounts the details of her 46th life as roaring-twenties party girl Grace Doze, hypnotherapy and real-life dovetail into a dramatic twist of fate. It was May 19, 1927, when the body of Grace Doze turned up in a Buffalo, N.Y., creek. Her murder remained a mystery until 60 years later, when Dr. Goldberg put Ivy into a superconscious state, and Grace's true killer was brought to light for the world to see.

1-56718-318-2, 6 x 9, 288 pp., photos, softcover   **$12.95**

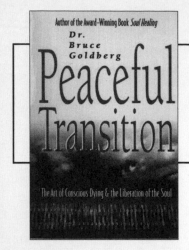

PEACEFUL TRANSITION
THE ART OF CONSCIOUS DYING & THE LIBERATION OF THE SOUL
Dr. Bruce Goldberg

Renowned past-life regression therapist Dr. Bruce Goldberg takes you on a journey like no other: that of letting go of your fear of death and facing it with a sense of honor and peace. He shows you the process of "conscious dying"—how to maintain a connection between your subconscious mind and your Higher Self at the moment of physical death in order to liberate yourself from the disorienting forces of the karmic cycle. To die without losing consciousness is at the very essence of immortality and enlightenment.

Peaceful Transition guides you in how to think, feel, and act before and during the moment of death. It presents actual case histories of patients who have successfully used these techniques, as well as exercises for you to use as a guide for your own transition.

1-56718-319-0, 6 x 9, 240 pp., softcover $12.95